# MENTAL HEALTH IN CHINA ⸺

# MENTAL HEALTH IN CHINA

Change, Tradition, and
Therapeutic Governance

Jie Yang

polity

First published in 2018 by Polity Press

Polity Press
65 Bridge Street
Cambridge CB2 1UR, UK

Polity Press
101 Station Landing
Suite 300,
Medford, MA 02155
USA

ISBN-13: 978-1-5095-0295-0
ISBN-13: 978-1-5095-0296-7 (pb)

A catalogue record for this book is available from the British Library.

Library of Congress Cataloging-in-Publication Data

Names: Yang, Jie, 1970- author.
Title: Mental health in China : psychologization and therapeutic governance / Jie Yang.
Description: Cambridge, UK; Malden, MA: Polity, 2017. | Series: China today | Includes bibliographical references and index.
Identifiers: LCCN 2017013935 (print) | LCCN 2017025905 (ebook) | ISBN 9781509502981(Mobi) | ISBN 9781509502998 (Epub) | ISBN 9781509502950 (hardback) | ISBN 9781509502967 (paperback)
Subjects: LCSH: Mental health--China. | Mental illness--China. | Mental health policy--China. | BISAC: MEDICAL / Mental Health.
Classification: LCC RA790.7.C6 (ebook) | LCC RA790.7.C6 Y36 2017 (print) | DDC 362.20951--dc23
LC record available at https://lccn.loc.gov/2017013935

Typeset in 11.5 on 15 pt Adobe Jenson Pro
by Toppan Best-set Premedia Limited
Printed and bound in Great Britain by CPI Group (UK) Ltd, Croydon

For further information on Polity, visit our website: politybooks.com

# Contents

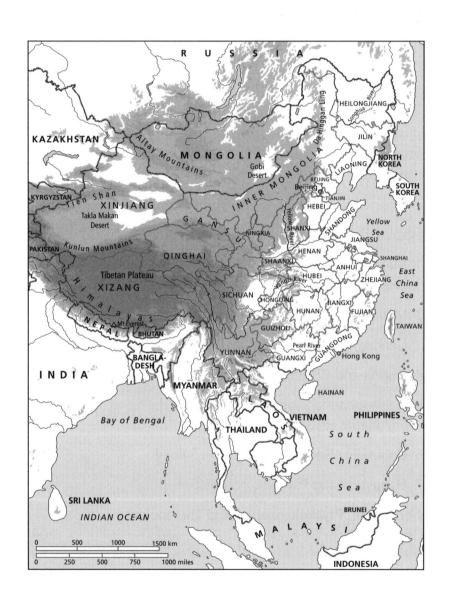

# Chronology

| | |
|---|---|
| 1894–5 | First Sino-Japanese War |
| 1898 | First mental health hospital established in Guangzhou, Guangdong Province, by American Medical Missionary John Kerr |
| 1911 | Fall of the Qing dynasty |
| 1912 | Republic of China established under Sun Yat-sen |
| 1917 | Institute of Psychology established in Beijing |
| 1927 | Split between Nationalists (KMT) and Communists (CCP); civil war begins |
| 1934–5 | CCP under Mao Zedong evades KMT in Long March |
| December 1937 | Nanjing Massacre |
| 1937–45 | Second Sino-Japanese War |
| 1945–9 | Civil war between KMT and CCP resumes |
| October 1949 | KMT retreats to Taiwan; Mao founds People's Republic of China (PRC) |
| 1950–3 | Korean War |
| 1953–7 | First Five-Year Plan; PRC adopts Soviet-style economic planning |
| 1954 | First constitution of the PRC and first meeting of the National People's Congress |
| 1956–7 | Hundred Flowers Movement, a brief period of open political debate |
| 1957 | Anti-Rightist Movement |
| 1958 | The first National Conference for Mental Illness Prevention in Nanjing |

| | |
|---|---|
| 1958–60 | The Great Leap Forward, an effort to transform China through rapid industrialization and collectivization |
| March 1959 | Tibetan Uprising in Lhasa; Dalai Lama flees to India |
| 1959–61 | Three Hard Years, widespread famine with tens of millions of deaths |
| 1960 | Sino-Soviet split |
| 1962 | Sino-Indian War |
| October 1964 | First PRC atomic bomb detonation |
| 1966–76 | Great Proletarian Cultural Revolution; Mao reasserts power |
| 1970 | The abolition of the Institute of Psychology, Chinese Academy of Sciences |
| February 1972 | President Richard Nixon visits China; "Shanghai Communiqué" pledges to normalize US–China relations |
| September 1976 | Death of Mao Zedong |
| October 1976 | Ultra-Leftist Gang of Four arrested and sentenced |
| December 1978 | Deng Xiaoping assumes power; launches Four Modernizations and economic reforms |
| 1978 | One-child family planning policy introduced |
| 1979 | US and China establish formal diplomatic ties; Deng Xiaoping visits Washington<br>PRC invades Vietnam<br>Mental Health Clinics opened at Beijing and Shanghai |
| 1982 | Census reports PRC population at more than one billion |
| December 1984 | Margaret Thatcher co-signs Sino-British Joint Declaration agreeing to return Hong Kong to China in 1997 |

| | |
|---|---|
| 1985 | Chinese Association for Mental Health established in Beijing |
| 1989 | Tiananmen Square protests culminate in June 4 military crack-down |
| 1992 | Deng Xiaoping's Southern Inspection Tour re-energizes economic reforms |
| 1993 | The inclusion of cultivating "psychological quality" in educational objectives by the Central Party policy |
| 1993–2002 | Jiang Zemin is president of PRC, continues economic growth agenda |
| 1997 | First Sino-German Mental Health Training Program started at Shanghai Mental Health Center |
| November 2001 | WTO accepts China as member |
| 2001 | National Mental Health License introduced by Ministry of Human Resources and Social Security |
| 2002–3 | SARS outbreak concentrated in PRC and Hong Kong |
| 2002–12 | Hu Jintao, General-Secretary of CCP (and President of PRC from 2003) |
| 2006 | PRC supplants US as largest $CO_2$ emitter |
| August 2008 | Summer Olympic Games in Beijing |
| 2008 | Psychological counselors aided victims from the Sichuan earthquake |
| 2010 | Shanghai World Exposition |
| 2012 | Xi Jinping appointed General-Secretary of the CCP (and President of PRC from 2013) First Mental Health Law of PRC |
| 2015 | National Mental Health Working Plan released by National Health and Family Planning Commission of PRC |

# Acknowledgements

I would like to thank all my informants and friends in both Beijing and Shandong Province for their generosity with their time, expertise, connections, and, most of all, for their trust. They opened so many doors for me to venture into diverse and multiple realms of mental health practices in China that compelled me to constantly rethink my research questions and expand my ethnographic inquiry. While I cannot thank them one by one publicly, their voices and insights permeate pages of the book. I hope that they like the way I interpreted their perspectives.

I presented materials drawn from this project at various conferences and institutions. I thank the organizers of and participants at these events: the annual meetings of the American Anthropological Association (2009–16); and the 2016 biannual meetings of the International Gender and Language Association, University of Victoria, University of Westminster, City University of Hong Kong, Free University Berlin, Columbia University, and Washington University at St. Louis. Special thanks go to Nick Bartlett, Anett Dippner, Derek Hird, Brian King, Daromir Rudnyckj, Julia Vorhoelter, and Gerda Wielander. I truly appreciate their valuable contributions to this book and treasure their friendship and support.

The book has benefited greatly from conversations with or written comments from Manduhai Buyandelger, Cherum Chu, Parin Dossa, Elsa Fan, Fang Yuanyuan, Zhipeng Gao, Lisa Hoffman, Hu Linying, Hu Xinying, Anru Lee, Ann-Marie Leshkowich, Mieke Matthyssen,

Carl Ratner, Pam Stern, Louise Sundararajan, Priscilla Song, Allen Tran, Wang Linan, Zhang Hong, Li Zhang, and Zhang Liao. I appreciate helpful research assistance from Marion Lougheed, Su Jing, and George Qingzhi Zhao. Janet Keller and Erin Martineau offered meticulous editorial guidance, intellectual inspiration, and helpful comments on the manuscript. I especially thank Marguerite Pigeon for her constant encouragement, support, and very insightful and valuable contributions to this project since 2014 when I started to draft the book.

I also benefited greatly from conversations and support from my colleagues at Simon Fraser University. Janice Matsumura has been a great mentor, and her constant encouragement and intellectual guidance have been extremely valuable over the years since I came to SFU. Barb Mitchell offered both extremely helpful insights on how to write a compelling book and important references. Robert Menzies at a crucial moment of this project offered encouragement and very helpful reference guidance. I thank him for being such a superb colleague, supportive mentor, and insightful scholar.

The data this book draws on were collected during field research for a big project on therapeutic governance in China funded by a multiyear standard research grant from the Social Sciences and Humanities Research Council of Canada. The final stage of writing was also supported by a Rapid Response Publication Grant from Simon Fraser University.

Writing this book would have been unimaginable without the trust of former editor at Polity Press Emma Longstaff, who first contacted me regarding this project in late 2014. I appreciate the way she contacted authors, personal, warm, and patient. Her insights into and guidance of the book proposal set the blueprint for the book. Jonathan Skerrett is a superb editor. I cannot thank him enough for all his help and labor. His clear and efficient guidance, thoughtful comments, and professionalism made it possible to bring this book to completion. Justin Dyer's meticulous and virtuosic editing is truly a gift. I thank

Justin and Neil de Cort for the great attention and care they gave to the manuscript. I also want to thank Nick Manning and the other anonymous reviewer for insightful comments and helpful suggestions, which were instrumental to my final revisions.

I dedicate this book to my mother, who passed away before its publication. In order not to distract me from my writing, she asked family members not to reveal her illness to me so that I dedicated my time to finish the book proposal in Vancouver in early 2015 before heading back to China. She made sure that I got in touch with a key research informant whom she had met through her doctor a few days before she was admitted to the Intensive Care Unit. My memory of her love, warmth, wisdom, and spiritual strength will nurture me and sustain me for the rest of my life.

# Introduction: China's Mental Health "Crisis"?    ————

> Work is therapy; without work, there is no way to talk about
> mental health.
> *A laid-off worker in Changping, Beijing*

> If it is those above who are sick, why are those at the bottom
> being fed the medicine?
> *A taxi-driver in Beijing*

> If you are addicted to work, you are praiseworthy, but if you are addicted to
> alcohol or the Internet, you are condemned; both involve similar
> psychological mechanisms of addiction. Psychology is moral judgment.
> *A psychological trainer in Beijing*

When considering China today from the outside, areas of concern
may include the environment, corruption, and the future of socialism.
Internally, however, these issues compete with another, more pressing
concern: mental illness. Chinese media and experts report that the
country is in the midst of a mental health "crisis" (Bi 2008; Chen 2010).
A 2009 survey by the Chinese Disease Control Center reported that
over 100 million of the 1.3 billion Chinese suffer some form of mental
illness (7.7 percent); within that group, over 16 million suffer severe
mental illness (Chen 2010) (16 percent). Compare this to the 1950s,
when the reported ratio of Chinese adults suffering from mental illness
was 1 in 37 (or 2.7 percent) (Yuen 2013). All told, about 190 million

Chinese are said to be in need of professional counseling or psychiatric treatment (Shao 2016) – a figure that exceeds the total in the 2009 survey above but one that aligns with global predictions: the World Health Organization estimates that by 2020 mental illness will account for one quarter of the overall health burden in China (Shao 2016).

China's mental health situation is exacerbated by a shortage of psychotherapeutic and psychiatric resources. Government support for mental health care is inadequate; current government spending for mental health accounts for less than 1 percent of total health expenditures (Qian 2012). China suffers from a lack of qualified doctors and of infrastructure such as wards and equipment (1,650 psychiatric facilities and a mere 15 psychiatric beds available for every 100,000 persons) (Zhang Jin 2016). There are 205,000 registered psychiatrists and 300,000 psychiatric nurses countrywide, equalling 1.49 psychiatrists per 100,000 people (Zhang Jin 2016). The doctor-to-patient ratio is 1:840, much lower than the world average (Liu 2016). Further, there are only 2.4 formally trained counselors for every 1 million people, in contrast with 3,000 per million in the United States (Han and Zhang 2007). As a result, about 92 percent of severely mentally ill Chinese do not receive treatment (Economist Intelligence Unit 2016: 10).[1]

These numbers paint a bleak picture. But instead of accepting statistics at face value, I want to go *through* them to reach the people in distress, as well as those offering them assistance, including psychiatrists, psychosocial workers, the state, and families. In this book, I use ethnography, media, and literature analysis to illuminate the experiences of these groups, and to discover how afflicted people, helpers, and the state interact to both create and alleviate the mental health "crisis." The central questions driving this exploration are: What has given rise to this mental health "crisis"? What are its characteristics and dynamics? And where will it lead in the future for millions of Chinese? I argue that the mental health "crisis" was mainly brought about by dislocation and rapid change amidst China's economic restructuring since the mid-1990s. Since then, the Chinese government has responded to this "crisis" by gradually integrating psychology into governance. This integration is intended not only to regulate alienated and confused subjects, but also to "empower" them, making them contributors to political stability and market development. The government orients this process towards achieving its political and economic interests by defining or manipulating basic human conditions, including happiness, well-being, sanity, normality, and gender identity. Far from departing from its single-party authority, the government mobilizes psychology and concepts of mental illness to resolve social, moral, economic, and political issues while legitimating the continued rule of the Communist Party.

The mental health "crisis" thus aligns psychology with the imperatives and needs of state and market. It creates and refashions forms of knowledge and spaces of interiority, which, however, because of their ambiguity, can be viewed by the government as sources of threats. This sometimes results in state responses based on fear: for instance, the case of Falun Gong.[2] The government has some reason to be concerned. The process of managing mental health in China indeed creates new forms of contestation and resistance. Overall, the domain of mental health is now used variously to support, contest, or grapple with power. The "crisis" also generates new forms of capital that bank on the suffering of millions, for example, leading to the booming counseling and psychopharmaceutical industry. Moreover, the "crisis" has revitalized elements of Chinese cultural tradition. The traditional Chinese notion of the heart, for example, has been increasingly highlighted and treated as an inner source of knowing, healing, value extraction, and contestation. With this emphasis on the heart – the basis of cognition, virtue, and bodily sensation (Ots 1994; Hall and Ames 1998) – Chinese psychological practices that are more embodied and holistic diverge from typically psyche-based Western psychology.

Since the 1980s, knowledge of Western psychotherapy, psychiatry, and psychopharmaceutical drugs has been steadily on the rise in China through globalization. This entry has given rise to new perceptions of suffering and well-being among Chinese people, and has brought new norms of healing and subjectivity. Thus, an ongoing dialectical interaction has emerged between Western psychological precepts and indigenous Chinese healing systems. In contrast to the Western dichotomy between the psyche and the body, in Chinese healing systems, the heart is the analytical core of diagnosis and treatment of mental illness. Instead of seeing illness as only endogenous to the person, Chinese therapeutic practices also draw attention to external causes of distress. In the current understanding of traditional healing, however, the external realm tends to be limited to intersubjective experiences, rather than structural or socioeconomic processes. In the following analysis, I emphasize some of these Chinese models of mental health care, which have much to offer the rest of the world, including novel perspectives on personhood and well-being that may provide new insights into mental health diagnostics and treatment. More generally, the mental health "crisis" offers new angles to think about consequences of social change and stratification and new ways of accessing resources and political reorientation.

In this book, I engage psychology not only as a knowledge system, but also as a cultural form – a culturally specific way of understanding and ordering actions (see Foucault 1998) – and as a way of thinking, imagining, and governing. By analyzing the use of psychology in guiding and regulating people and everyday life, I examine the complex, multilayered relationships between socioeconomic development, governance, and subjectivity that have shaped China since Mao's era. Using psychology as a technique of power, the state, in its effort to tighten control, can actually create the appearance of conceding power. It is a form of governance that works through "care" more than force. The Chinese government both "cares" for its people and mobilizes them to care for themselves through psychological means; the focus on psychological and personal care also diverts attention from social and economic processes that could spark criticism of the state.

## "SUBHEALTH" IN A "HARMONIOUS SOCIETY"

Since the mid-1990s, many Chinese state-owned enterprises have been restructured or privatized. These economic transformations have driven an all-consuming search for wealth, as well as changes in communal and family structures, as millions of rural people have migrated to cities for jobs. Many Chinese are experiencing these changes as traumatic. The work-unit system that once provided a lifelong institutional basis for material and emotional support (Walder 1986) has been gradually dismantled, and urban workers must now turn to family and friends for this help. However, the efficacy of informal support as the primary form of welfare is questionable. For example, migrant workers, most of whom live far from home, often do not have reliable friends nearby, and have nowhere to turn for psychological and material support.[3] It is this structural lack that psychology, the government, self-help projects, and therapeutic consumption attempt to address.

In a book titled *Where the Anxiety of Chinese Came From* (2013), Mao Yushi analyzes sources of anxiety and distress among Chinese people, including social injustice, rising housing prices, widening income gaps, the stark privileges of certain groups, poverty, employment difficulties, food safety, the exam-centered educational system, and environmental contamination. To some, such sources of anxiety contribute to widespread *ya jiankang*, or "subhealth," in the country (Liu 2008; Bunkenborg 2014; Yang 2017). Subhealth is a specific state of distress, a compromised position of ambiguity and insecurity between health and illness that manifests itself psychologically and somatically. Though not a diagnostic category, it is often invoked by doctors to describe undesirable physical and psychological conditions that, without attention, may develop into disease. Subhealth reportedly affects about 80 percent of the Chinese population (Liu 2008). Middle-aged Chinese, facing double pressure from both children and aging parents, reportedly suffer more subhealth, but all age groups seem to be more vulnerable to subhealth now than in the past.

Anxiety, instability, and subhealth jar with and even defy the goals of China's political project of constructing a "harmonious society," as envisioned by Hu Jintao and Wen Jiabao in 2004. The harmonious society is characterized by vitality as well as democracy, the rule of law, equity, justice, sincerity, and amity. To narrow the gap between social distress and imagined social harmony, the Chinese government has taken action – but not really focusing on the structural features of life, including jobs and social support. Rather, together with psychological and psychiatric (psy) experts, it has made efforts to individualize, internalize, and psychologize the social, moral, and political issues that generate conflicts, perplexities, moral confusion, and illnesses.

## "PSYCHOBOOM": THE GROWING MENTAL HEALTH INDUSTRY

With mental illness now firmly on the list of national health concerns, researchers, medical practitioners, and drug companies are developing new initiatives to tackle the issue, thereby promoting the rapid development of China's mental health industry.[4] Legal frameworks have been established to accommodate this growth. In October 2012, the National People's Congress passed a mental health law safeguarding patients' medical privacy and prohibiting involuntary treatment. In its 13th Five-Year Plan (2016–20) the Chinese government also promised to enhance investment in and support for mental health care, especially at the grassroots level. Most recently, in early 2017, the first guideline on improving mental health in China was issued by 22 ministries and departments. According to this guideline, the state will promote mental health education and awareness across China by 2020, increase access to mental health services, and enhance the general level of people's mental health by 2030 (Wang 2017).

This is the context for China's current "psychoboom" – the awakening interest in counseling, psychology books, psychological idioms of distress, psychometric methods, and psychotherapy training (Kleinman 2010: 1075; see also Yang 2013; Huang 2014; L. Zhang 2014). More people are now coming into contact with psychiatrists and therapists – some in person, but most through books, films, online, and in popular discourse. Tropes derived from this psychological discourse permeate television shows, online programs, and everyday life. The self-help industry has also flourished. Counseling or therapy becomes, to some extent, entertainment or leisure. Online counseling, like the popular "Psychology Talk Show" airing on China Central Television (CCTV), has moved talk therapy from private counseling rooms to public screens, making "confessing one's personal problems ... a subject of mass entertainment" (Moskowitz 2001: 246). Meanwhile, the Ministry of Civil Affairs and Ministry of Labour offer psychological training to human resource management personnel, community workers, and employee assistance program (EAP) counselors. Since 2009, psychological health has become an important criterion when selecting Chinese cadres and officials (Shao 2016).

While the psychoboom promotes awareness of individual rights and could de-stigmatize mental health issues, many counselors offer poor guidance, often over-applying psychological theories that do not take into account the unique Chinese context. For example, following Western psychologists, Chinese counselors have recently begun attributing psychological issues to early childhood trauma. Yet Chinese cultural perspectives highlight the positive effect of suffering on child development, as captured in the sayings "*jia pin chu xiaozi*" (poor family produces respectful children) and "*bu jing yi shi, bu zhang yi zhi*" (wisdom grows with failures or difficulties). Focusing on individual trauma alone is also reductive given that, in the Chinese context, emotions are viewed as socially produced. Thus, the psychotherapeutic practices in China tend to adopt a narrower lens on suffering than traditional wisdom, often excluding exogenous sources of distress.

## PSYCHOLOGIZATION IN THE REFORM ERA: FROM SOCIALISM AND THE STATE TO THE SELF

The psychoboom or psychologization trend is concurrent with a gradual depoliticization of social life and growing emphasis on the self in China (Kleinman et al. 2011; Kipnis 2012). Psychologization is the medicalization of mental health, where the idea of disease or illness is deployed to make sense of conditions and experiences that are distinctly social and cultural. It uses psychological knowledge or biomedical rationality to deal with social issues. In general, three modes of psychologization have emerged in China. First is the popularization by both the state and the public of psychological labels, psychological explanatory schemes, and psychological modes of thinking that result in widespread informal diagnoses. The overflow of psychological discourse has created new mental and psychological "illnesses," including "road rage," "unemployment complex syndrome," "officials' heartache," and "Internet addiction," all of which provide a medical or psychological label that interprets social experiences (see Chapter 2). A second mode has resulted in increased emphasis on *xinli hua*: reasoning by and into the heart. *Xinli hua* refers to the process of understanding others and the world from the perspective of the heart (Han 2016). This involves empathically looking at the "heart" or nature of the person or situation, thereby engaging intersubjective experience; it is based on the Chinese notion that the heart is more fundamental to being than the body. The third mode of psychologization has led to the entanglement of psychological rhetoric and tactics with power mechanisms and the market. This entanglement turns social, economic, and political issues into domains suitable for psychological intervention, and diverts public attention from broader social processes toward individual inadequacies, masking government culpability for abetting mental distress.

Psychologization has impacted mental health care in China. Today, the government and psy experts, as well as ordinary people and those who suffer psychological disorders, draw on a mix of Western psychotherapy and Chinese cultural tradition. As Jyrki Kallio writes, "[T]radition and history have become the Chinese communist party's tools of choice for bolstering its legitimacy. The party is attempting to patch the chinks in its rusting spiritual-ideological armor with a concoction of handpicked values from traditional schools of thought, especially Confucianism" (2011: 1). Indeed, Confucian political values and the Confucian notion of the self with collective ambience have been increasingly invoked in China since the 1990s (Shi 2015).[5] If in the West the psychotherapist constructs and cares for interiority, in China, by invoking cultural traditions, psychotherapists collaborate with the state to care for and to govern both the spaces of interiority and ensemble or relational selves. This mixed genre of healing resources makes psychologization pervasive, subtle, and hegemonic.

## PSYCHO-POLITICS: RECONFIGURING THE INNER SELF

The mental health "crisis" partially results from and contributes to changing configurations of the self and subjectivity in China's reform era (since 1978). Amidst mass socioeconomic dislocation, the state, together with psy experts, seeks to construct and regulate new types of subjects who are more mobile and self-reliant. During the early years of reform (1980s–90s), the bigger world was still largely unknown. Leaving the public sector for the private market was deemed *xia hai*, literally meaning "going down to the sea," like a plunge into the unknown. Three decades of market adventure later, many have mastered the ropes. What remains is an inner wilderness: the interior of the self. China's market development is implicitly depicted as an aggressive, heartless movement. Interiority becomes the opposite: a new frontier for healing spiritual emptiness and moral confusion. While this interiority may point to new possibilities, it is hidden and mysterious and viewed widely as potentially subversive; interiority thus becomes a new site for (governmental) scrutiny and intervention.

Unlike the empty self predominantly characterized by absence in the post-World War II United States (Cushman 1992), the new, reform-era Chinese self is seen as excessive – overrun by desires, values, and feelings, which unsettle the heart. To achieve peace, the self must be purged and filled up anew with whatever could bring meaning, certainty, and identity. Today, psychology and psychotherapy are therefore involved in healing this overfull self. What is left unsaid, however, is the extent to which they create this self, especially among the middle class and elites. For the working class and marginalized groups, the self is constructed somewhat differently; it tends to be imputed as angry and dangerous for men, or happy and productive for women (see J. Yang 2015). In general, the Chinese state emphasizes social stability and market development, acting as both guarantor of an entrepreneurial (but anxious, desirous) middle-class self and controller of a (demoralized) working-class self that is full of restless and dangerous impulses.

In some ways, this political concern with people's inner selves is continuous with Mao's era. During the Cultural Revolution (1966–76), the population was mobilized to spy on one another and report ideas that deviated from Maoist ideologies. People were forced to use set formulae and fixed expressions from Mao's works in an effort to frame their consciousness and ensure political conformity (Ji 2004). To some extent, the widespread psychological discourse in today's China provides a new language for people to make sense of their experience of socioeconomic dislocation. But unlike Mao – a master narrator transmitting his ideologies to the masses through linguistic engineering – current psychological discourse is diffuse, often disseminated by diverse sources through varied rhetoric and methods, with an appeal to feelings, or through a self-help logic adapted from both the West and the Chinese tradition of self-cultivation. Unlike the condemnation of self-centeredness in Mao's era, current psychological discourses encourage individuals to retreat into their private and inner lives. Social "deviance" is now more pathologized than politicized. Whereas in Mao's time, mental problems were attributed to obsessively selfish ideas and personal concerns (Munro 2002) that the state could cure through public ideological re-education, today psychological technologies not only enable individuals to promote self-reflection and self-governance, but also equip governments and institutions to delve into a person's heart, emotions, capacities, and intimate relationships.

The incidence of mental illness today arises from multiple factors, especially market reform and destruction of the community orientation of socialist ethics. This would be a crisis under most circumstances, but inadequate social services and political priorities exacerbate the situation. The mental health "crisis" also relates to Party-oriented political institutions that, confronted with economic and political pressures, have sought to maintain authority and legitimacy in changing times. The creation and governing of new interiorities, for example through psychology, thus plays a significant role in China's political and economic restructuring. However, while offering optimism, hope, and the promise of happiness, health, and success, psychology, as presently employed, manipulates people's perception of social reality. A new form of politics has emerged based on this use of psychology to govern spaces of interiority, including the heart, subconsciousness, the inner child, and human potential (see Chapter 6). I call this "psycho-politics," which governs the heart and inner life, resembling biopolitics, which inscribes power on the body (Foucault 1978). However, in psycho-politics, the body and the heart are treated not only as a site of power inscription but also as forces that converge and transduce social, political, and economic forces. Here I exemplify this point by focusing on the heart as a force in Chinese psychology.

The heart has many functions, chief of which is to provide a moral core for subjectivity and agency. This core is necessary to achieve equanimity, a state of equilibrium in which one is not shaken by external disturbances. In this state, spontaneous bodily reactions are regulated by the heart's high moral reflection. For this reason, Chinese psychotherapists adopt a socio-moral approach to mental illness, rather than viewing it as purely personal pathology or neurochemical imbalance (see also Kleinman 1986). In addition, the heart has epistemological functions. It is forever observing itself, wondering about its true nature, agonizing over what it hides and ways of controlling bodily impulses, and reckoning with one's potential and limits. The knowledge produced by the heart has been historically viewed as more authentic than that produced purely by the mind (see *xinli hua* above). This understanding of the heart seems to collapse the boundary between reason and emotion and between soma and psyche. We can see how this heart epistemology can be amenable to governance – the heart cares about the inner and interpersonal life. The state can therefore promote independent interiorities and self-absorption, confining individual attention to intersubjective realms rather than broader social processes, preventing large-scale collective protest even in times of crisis.

## THERAPEUTIC GOVERNANCE AND SUBJECTIVITY

The trend of psychologization is partly enabled by a shift toward what can be called "therapeutic governance," or an increasing attention within governments to the ideas, languages, and practices of therapeutic expertise (Pupavac 2001, 2005). As mental illnesses are not simply diseases, but also social and cultural constructs (Foucault 1976), idioms of distress (Nichter 2010), or "syndromes" of common experiences, including physical sensations, moral order, and social interactions (Good 1977), this mode of therapeutic governing is reductive and homogenizing. Within this mode, mental illness becomes an amenable conceptual tool entangled with economic and political practices and manipulated as a way of allocating resources, and is thus inevitably a source of critique and contestation.

Vanessa Pupavac (2001) defines therapeutic governance as a mode of control through which psychosocial intervention is used to manage social risk. Pupavac notes that while engendered in the Anglo-American context, this form of governance has spread to the global South via Western hegemony. It resembles Foucault's notion of governmentality, which relies on particular practices of observing, monitoring, shaping, or controlling the behaviors of individuals (Gordon 1991). Therapeutic governance can be described as an art of governing through the dissemination of therapeutic expertise, psychological knowledge, or biomedical rationality in society. This type of governance is underpinned by the assumptions that therapeutic methods can improve psychological health and doing so is part of good governance, and that it is in government's and society's best interest to protect and improve individual psychological well-being.

However, while in Western literature, psy experts play a key role in governmentality (Rose 1996; Miller and Rose 2008; Matza 2012) and the therapeutic state (Szasz 1963; Polsky 1991; Nolan 1998), in China, psy experts are dispensable. Therapeutic governance can be carried out by non-medical agencies and institutions (Chen 2010), or even the public through popular psychological imagination and informal diagnosis. This non-medical practice is partly a lingering effect of Maoist perceptions of mental illness as social or ideological pathology, or partly a product of the capricious, sovereign power of the Chinese state. For instance, in the case of suicides among Chinese officials, the government accepts informal diagnoses by media and employers that blame the deaths on biomedical depression, thus bypassing medical authorities – a move that serves its own need for expediency and limited scrutiny of the bureaucracy.[6] Such informal diagnosis can be applied to dead bodies (of those officials who committed suicide), part of China's broader necropolitics: the state has the authority to define life and death, control dead bodies, and interpret the causes of deaths (cf. Mbembe 2003). Informal diagnosis may also flow from traditional practices of health and well-being in Chinese society, which rely on self-cultivation in nurturing life (Farquhar and Zhang 2012). With enough exposure to the media and government-sponsored training, anyone can become a mental health "expert."

Therapeutic governance is both a result of the post-socialist transformation and a response to widespread stress and emotional and moral disorientation resulting from privatization and marketization since the mid-1990s (see J. Yang 2015 and Zhang 2017 on different modes of Chinese therapeutic governance). Uncertainty and stress among citizens about the rules and norms of governing life have created a demand for psychological answers. The state responds to the demand in part through therapeutic paradigms: addressing public life via the psychoboom (Kleinman 2010), tackling family issues through marriage counseling and the professionalization of parenting (Kuan 2015), and managing effects of economic restructuring such as heroin addiction and unemployment through psychotherapeutic interventions (J. Yang 2015; Bartlett 2016). By popularizing psychological knowledge, the government and the public may invest it with ideological and ethical contents, turning knowledge into a mode of regulation and control. Further, imbuing diverse social domains with a therapeutic ethos shifts the focus from practices informed by Marxist materialism and social reality to heart-based practices informed by psychology, which rely on narratives and interpretive stances rather than on "objective" reality (see Illouz 2008). The new locus of agency is the heart (or interiority) – a venue for knowledge production, a nexus of cultural expression, a mode of self-management, and a target of both power and contestation.

What results is more hegemonic forms of power in which the state/ therapist approaches its people/clients through "care" and "permissive empathy" (Parsons 1965), or through psychological discourses that shape the public's imagination. Unlike previous psychiatric attempts to improve narrowly defined social domains and functions – for example, in the treatment of political dissidents in Mao's era (Munro 2002) – psychologization today suffuses a wide range of institutions, practices, and discourses. While un- or under-diagnosis has been a serious issue in China owing to limited mental health care resources, within this hegemonic presence of psychology many people are subject to over-diagnosis or misdiagnosis, or even mislabeled as mentally ill. In my research, I learned of a woman named Xu Xueling who was twice forcibly hospitalized for being "hysterical," despite a lack of any supporting formal diagnosis (see Chapter 1). She had petitioned her local government to contest the leniency granted to an employee of Xinwen Mining Company in Shandong Province who had seriously injured her sister. The government defied its own mental health law by opportunistically "diagnosing" and forcibly hospitalizing Xu in order to discredit her legal claim. The case illustrates that therapeutic governance in China encompasses both sovereign components through medical and institutional control and more hegemonic forms of regulation through psychological "care" or psychological imagination.

Xu's case also hints at how psychological techniques are enmeshed with welfare networks to govern vulnerable individuals and groups. Unlike the Western therapeutic (welfare) state, which tends to normalize marginalized people to minimize the role of the state in the lives of individuals (Polsky 1991), psychological "care" offered through China's poverty relief and re-employment programs *nurtures* angry, despondent members of disadvantaged groups (men in particular) to appease them and sustain stability. These processes highlight the "benevolence" of the state, transforming the poor from subjects with rights to objects of care, and translating the exercise of power into affective and therapeutic activities (J. Yang 2013, 2015). By embracing therapeutic practices and ideologies, power can operate at a distance. As Peter Miller and Nikolas Rose point out, this translation leads to "therapeutic authority," which "poses in a new way, an old problem in the exercise of authority – the relation between authority over others and authority over the self" (1994: 36). It is not a repressive force; rather it is more akin to a new style of thought, "endowing individuals with new competencies, aptitudes and qualities" (1994: 36). Indeed, while Western therapeutic governing posits the self as fragile, requiring continuous therapeutic guidance (Furedi 2004; Pupavac 2005), therapeutic governing in China also promotes a positive vision of realizing human potential particularly through precepts of positive psychology, "positive energy" (see Chapter 7), and positive values of Chinese cultural tradition (J. Yang 2015).

In Western studies of therapeutic governance, the emphasis on the power of experts more than on those who are subject to psy power fails to fully demonstrate the effects of psychologization on individuals – the degree of the intrusiveness of Western biomedicine into individual minds and bodies – and elides the agency and contestation of those subject to psy expertise. This elision may also foreclose alternative, indigenous sources of healing or communal practices of coping with the consequences of violence or socioeconomic dislocations. My work diverges from these Western frameworks by considering the role of culture and phenomenology in the study of therapeutic governance. Specifically, I highlight the theoretical and methodological importance of focusing on individual voices and lived experiences with psy power.

Indeed, therapeutic governance centers on the management of subjectivity. Psychology has provided people with new concepts through which to conceive themselves and the world, as well as with techniques of care, healing, and self-fashioning. As individuals are "made up"

(Hacking 1986) through psychology (often endorsed by the government in China), their subjectivity can ally with and reproduce state interests.

Embracing therapeutics has also helped the state forge new points of contact with the public and to recoup a less antagonistic relationship between governors and governed in China. Talcott Parsons (1965) pointed out that while other institutional interventions can leave individual subjectivity untouched, therapy brings with it the possibility of influencing people's internal lives. Indeed, suffering is the very link between therapists and patients. Rather than judge or moralize their suffering or behaviors, therapists empathize with the individuals and establish a sense of "permissiveness" with them (Parsons 1965: 317). Through such permissive empathy, therapists can gain privileged access to people's subjectivity. They are also able to reward compliance through providing individuals with a diagnosis.

In the wake of rapid social change, therapeutic governance in China is part of state efforts to solidify political legitimacy. It seems to constitute the state efforts to implement the Confucian doctrine of *minben*, emphasizing the moral aim of government as benefiting the people. However, the ultimate aim of *minben* is actually to keep the rulers in power (Shi and Lu 2010a). Since traditional China, people have judged the performance of the state not merely in terms of its economic performance, but also in terms of how well it has dealt with crises. Today, various state efforts, including passing the first Mental Health Law in 2012, advocating for community-based mental health care, and the alleged increase in financial investment in mental health, show that the government attempts to continue bolstering its legitimacy through management of the mental health "crisis." Further, these therapeutic efforts contribute to *xianneng zhengzhi*, or "political meritocracy," a political system that relies on morally superior and capable leaders governing for the people (Bell 2015). Psychological "care" for the people highlights the role of the state as people's "guardian," part of the

Party's "guardian discourse," contributing to its legitimacy (Shi and Lu 2010b).

In addition to guardianship, the Chinese government has played varying roles in mental health care. For example, it carefully cultivates the positive potential of "negative" emotions such as anger or anxiety to enhance the productivity and entrepreneurship of white-collar workers for market development while it pathologizes and condemns the anger and restlessness of the working class (especially men) to sustain sociopolitical stability. Rather than a heavy-handed top-down approach to mental health, the government deploys multiple powers: disciplinary, biopolitical, necropolitical, stigmatic, and therapeutic, both sovereign and hegemonic.

## COMMERCIALIZING MENTAL DISTRESS

China's mental health woes have contributed to rapidly developing mental health and wellness industries, including private mental hospitals, vast self-help genres, commercialized counseling, and the popularity of psychopharmaceutical drugs. Taking advantage of the niche market created by the limited public mental health services, more and more private mental facilities, such as the well-known Kangning Hospital (recently listed in the Hong Kong stock market), have been established to offer psychiatric treatment for millions in China. Since 2015, at least 10 psychological counseling companies have received venture-fund investment; four of these have stock values exceeding 100 million yuan. The Internet has also enabled this market to grow exponentially (by over 30 times). Chinese psychology is mostly practiced online through the immensely popular Chinese phone app WeChat. In search of profit, many psychotherapists now focus more on group training for white-collar workers in big corporations, or online group counseling, than one-on-one private talk therapy. Psychotherapy has been integral to China's market economy.

Meanwhile, the widespread anxiety, loneliness, and alienation in China have also spurred new businesses such as *peiban jingji*, the "companion economy." Websites and (online) "shops" have been set up to help clients cope with their negative emotions including anger, loneliness, sadness, or shyness, through delivering them congratulations, apologies, empathy, offering them anger management or bed-warming services,[7] and finding clients marriage partners or surrogate girlfriends or boyfriends for holiday seasons to avoid parental nagging.[8] New professions such as *peiliao*, "companionable counselors" or "chatting companions," have also emerged to help people cope with distress and suffering. In Changping, Beijing, companionable counseling to those who are lonely, sick, and distressed has been mainly performed by laid-off-women-workers-turned-housemaids or rural-migrants-turned-domestic-workers (see J. Yang 2015).

Further, advertising now uses psychological techniques to sell products and services, linking commodities with particular states of being. Such advertising implies that through "consuming" a certain commodity, the consumer's identity will become transformed; by using a product or ingesting a drug, one expects to achieve the health and lifestyle of the model featured in the advertisement (Ewen 1989). Commodities thus become transformational objects, and consumption becomes a transformative and therapeutic process. Such therapeutic consumption targets particularly those who suffer subhealth, a state of ambiguity or moral confusion. In general, within this trend of psychologization, ambiguous interiority and the heart can become (new) sites and resources for value extraction and entrepreneurial capital.

## RESEARCH METHODOLOGY AND CHAPTER SUMMARY

I have conducted multi-sited ethnographic research on the mental health of underprivileged, elite, and middle-class groups in China since

2002. While focusing my fieldwork on the psychological and emotional effects of state-enterprise restructuring on workers in Changping, Beijing, since 2009, I have paid particular attention to the mental health of unemployed workers and state-led psychotherapeutic interventions in Beijing, and have followed community psychosocial workers during training sessions. When attending training sessions on counseling, EAP, social work, and self-help, I have interviewed instructors and other psychosocial workers, as well as laid-off-women-workers-turned-*peiliao* (chatting companions) from different districts of Beijing and Zhangqiu, Shandong Province.

During the summers of 2009–13, and over three months in 2015, I conducted participant observation and interviews at two Chinese mental hospitals: one in Changping deemed MKH, which is sponsored by the Chinese Ministry of Civil Affairs and serves mainly vulnerable groups; the other a mental health center, ZYH, in Zhangqiu that operates as a wing of a general hospital. I usually split my summers between both hospitals. At both locations I spoke with psychiatrists and nurses about the patterns and treatment of psychiatric disorders, and with patients and their families about their illness experiences and treatment alternatives. While working as a research intern at MKH and ZYH, I analyzed patient records, epidemiological data, and ward surveys, from which I developed case studies for this project. I have also followed many patients I met at the two hospitals to their homes and conducted in-depth household interviews with them and their family members. I labeled these data, for example, MKH/ZYH-2009 (year of the first interview)-d(doctor)2 (roughly indicating the order of my first interview with this psychiatrist among all the psychiatrists I have interviewed in that hospital, even though I might have interviewed them multiple times over the years). Similarly, in-/outpatients I interviewed at length on wards or at home are the basis for the book's case studies. These are labeled, for example, MKH/ZYH-2010-p (patient)11. When citing interviews with counselors and psychiatrists outside MKH or ZYH, I use, for example, BJ (Beijing)-2013 (year of first interview)-c(counselor)23/d(psychiatrist)21.

During my research, some of my former classmates and childhood friends in Zhangqiu, where I grew up, and who are now middle-ranking officials, asked for my help in being referred to psychiatrists in Beijing. This experience compelled me to initiate a research project in 2009 on the mental health of lower-level officials – the so-called *guan xinbing*, "officials' heartache" – in Zhangqiu. My friendships or acquaintances with these subjects have opened many new doors for me to access the grassroots bureaucracy, which enriched my work tremendously. Given the reportedly increased rates of depression and suicide among Chinese officials since 2013, this project is crucial to understanding the sociopolitical etiology of mental illness.[9]

The first four chapters of the book map mental health, mental illness, and psychologization in China, their interactions with class and gender dimensions, and the stigma associated with mental illness. The final three chapters track the development of psychology and its cognates in China, including psychiatry, counseling, indigenous psychology, and self-help.

In Chapter 1, I review Chinese concepts of mental health and illness, highlighting contradictions and conflicts in illness categories and treatment practices, including views of social versus biological roots of distress. I emphasize the impacts of psychiatric treatment on the growing mental health industry and political stabilization. In Chapter 2, I study the multiplying new mental "illnesses" in the context of China's psychoboom, including "smog depression/blues," "Internet addiction," "princess disease," "empty-heart disease," and "petitioning addiction/petitioning bigotry," and consider how political and social "deviance" and differences have been psychologized, and to what ends. Next, Chapter 3 observes important gender- and class-based differences in the definition, distribution, and treatment of mental disorders, and how the Chinese state utilizes these differences for its own social, economic, and political purposes. Through analysis of the discourse pathologizing "unhappy" and "depressed" mothers and the "sick-man phenomenon," I highlight a trend toward essentialization that abets social exclusion and exploitation of women. Chapter 4 focuses on the stigma associated with mental illness. I show that stigma acts as both an informal mode of control and a mode of governing. Alternatively, stigma can become a means for those who suffer from mental illness and their families to manipulate and optimize mental illness for their own benefit.

Chapter 5 turns to psychiatric hospital care and psychopharmacological practices. Drawing on ethnographic examples at two mental hospitals, I challenge the often reductive psychopharmacological approaches taken in hospital-based psychiatric practice in China. My analysis shows that despite the tendency for blanket pharmacological solutions to foreclose unique experiences of distress, mental patients and their family members can negotiate and contest this treatment approach and its side-effects and expand patients' subjectivities. In Chapter 6, I look closely at the integration of Western and indigenous psychologies. The chapter unfolds the classist orientation of various therapies grafting precepts of Confucianism, Daoism, and Buddhism onto Western psychotherapy and reveals that while the refinement and hybridity of Western and indigenous psychologies addresses citizens' needs in a time of transformation, they can also mask an avenue for state influence in self-development. Finally, Chapter 7 examines China's vast self-help genre, or *xinling jitang* (chicken soup for the soul) and the promotion of happiness. As part of the psychoboom, *xinling jitang* captures psychology's "overflow" into the broader realms of society and its entanglement with power mechanisms. The analysis focuses on how *xinling jitang* is co-opted via state-led happiness campaigns and the official promotion of *zheng nengliang* (positive energy) to achieve social, economic, and political objectives and to cultivate happy, productive, and moral subjects.

Taken together, these chapters delineate a set of changes, political and therapeutic practices, and lived experiences that characterize China's mental health "crisis." Partly an opportunity for the state to expand markets, control the population, and authorize itself, and partly a real experience of distress among Chinese people and their attempts to grapple with profound historical, social, and economic change, the mental health "crisis" is neither an invention nor simply a matter of ailing hearts. It is a window that allows us to see China's uneven development as an emerging major power, its shifting governance, and their effects on its people and their well-being and subjectivity.

# 1 Mental Health and Mental Illness: Concepts and Contradictions

> Mental health is having enough to eat and a good sleep at night.
> *A taxi-driver in Beijing*

> If one has *bentou* [something to strive for] in life, one won't get depressed or commit suicide.
> *A male worker at Changping*

Still today, mental distress in China is often attributed to weakness or foreign influence. Such views may derive from Mao's era, when private life and personal problems were moralized or politicized, and mental illness was often stigmatized as attitude problems caused by ill-advised ideological positions emerging from bourgeois capitalism, or as "thought diseases" resulting from diminished revolutionary zeal (Munro 2002). During the Cultural Revolution, many mentally ill patients were taken from hospitals and sent to labor camps because of their "counterrevolutionary" behavior (Munro 2002). The view of mental distress as a political evil or as social and ideological pathology more than a disease may have hindered the development of local forms of psychiatry, psychotherapy, or other integrative healing techniques, but it assisted in bringing about some of the unique forms of psychological practice in China today.

Nowadays, "deviants" or "dissidents" are no longer judged prejudicially as being on the extreme political right or left, as counterrevolutionary, or as antipatriotic. They are deemed sick or mad and in need of medical or therapeutic intervention. Mental health is generally appreciated as an integral part of one's overall well-being. In my interviews, Chinese counselors referred to health as including not only psychological well-being, but also holistic health integrating the body and the heart. They tended to accept medical authority and advise clients to follow doctors' diagnoses and prescriptions and to face disease bravely. Such pluralism is characteristic of the practices of psychology that have evolved in China during the recent psychoboom. These counselors themselves offer physical exercises and prescribe a positive attitude to combat depression, anxiety, and other mental distress. They ask clients to pay attention to nutrition and diet to cultivate health and nurture life. They recommend a peaceful and balanced heart, the moral core of one's subjectivity, together with a moving body as key to health and longevity (Hao 2014). Mental health means freedom not only from psychological and psychiatric problems but also from moral confusion. In general, for counselors in Beijing, health is not only body-heart-spirit integration, an acceptance of one's self, and an avenue that channels efficient energy, but it is also a personal choice and an active lifestyle. Yet even as health is viewed in the Chinese context holistically as a whole-body-mind-spirit concept, a more individualized Western biomedicine continues to be widely adopted and Chinese psychiatrists emphasize biomedical treatment of symptoms rather than redressing societal impetuses for distress. The ultimate resolution to mental illness remains the call for clients to adapt to the social environment by readjusting their values and attitudes and reconstructing their cognition.

Traditional Chinese wisdom and practices for health and well-being rely on the self – a vague, fluid sense of being in social networks. The culture of self-cultivation has been encouraged in recent decades by the government in the hope that people will manage the challenges required to cope with reduced state welfare support as a result of privatization and economic restructuring (see Farquhar and Zhang 2012). There is a sense that everyone should become a health "expert," taking care of themselves. The self, defined relationally as part of the familial and social network, anticipates the social resources that individuals need to deal with anxiety and stress, thus cushioning the impact of social and economic struggles that derive from state-led economic restructuring while preventing people from directly confronting the government. Such relational support comes in both emotional and material forms: networks provide not only ways to channel complaints and grievances internally without needing to reach out to criticize the government but also temporary material support for those who are economically impoverished, for example as a result of layoffs (J. Yang 2015).

The concept of mental health in China is influenced by Confucian ideology as well as an emphasis on family. In contrast to Western thought, the Chinese emphasize "personal duties and social goals" rather than individual rights (Hsiao et al. 2006). Indeed, the ideal Chinese self is rooted in its value for society (Fei 1992). Failing to fulfill one's duties within the family and society can be unsettling and lead to symptoms of mental distress, such as feelings of guilt and shame. Interpersonal harmony is key to maintaining mental health and well-being (Hsiao et al. 2006). In a Confucian milieu, (mental) health is dealt with in everyday life through living up to one's responsibilities toward others. Health concerns oneself, but oneself is realized through the ties with family: loved ones, parents, children, brothers, and sisters. Similar to the definition of mental health that circulates in other East Asian countries like Japan (Lock 1993; Borovoy 2005; Kitanaka 2012), mental health or distress in China has often been viewed as a form of sociomoral experience (Kleinman 1986; Lee and Kleinman 2003) impacted by social and cultural factors (Kleinman 1980, 1986; Bond 1986).

Mental health in China must be understood not only by taking into account Confucian influence, but also in the context of modern history. Indeed, history has played a role in defining the forms of mental distress. As a nation, China experienced turmoil over the idea of "catching up with the West," which began at the end of the Opium Wars (1839–42) (Zhou 2014), creating a sense of crisis and anxiety for individuals. More recently, amidst China's tumultuous transition from a socialist planned economy to a market economy, widespread socio-economic dislocation has also caused ubiquitous anxiety and stress.

Further, given the relational and embodied view of psychology in China, the construction of personhood clashes with Western individualism and particular biomedical techniques of psychiatry. Western psychotherapy may prove detrimental in China as a result of a poor fit with the relational senses of the self. However, a new political culture in China is emerging based on neoliberal economic entrepreneurship of the self, as is a new psychological culture founded on atomization of subjectivities, and their independence constitutes selfhood for the Chinese middle class. But the working class remains outside this new paradigm, straddling Mao's self-formation (in which the self was interdependently linked with others and with work units) and the current call for individuality based on self-reliance.

Current (governmental) reliance on individual psychology and biomedical rationale to account for structurally induced distress – that is, psychologization – can influence various facets of personhood including desire, enterprise, and morality recently explored by anthropologists (Rofel 2007; Zhang and Ong 2008; Kleinman et al. 2011). The goal for the Chinese state appears to create ideal, happy subjects who do not rock the boat politically, who are psychologically obsessive but politically inactive. But there are gaps, inconsistencies, and disruptions that mar the government's plan for "optimal" self-formation.

By destabilizing psychological metanarratives and emphasizing distinctions among conceptualizations of madness along with the economic, legislative, religious, and ethical factors in the regulation of the mad that predominate during different historical eras, Foucault (1976) suggests that both the form and etiology of madness must be sought not in the body or psyche, but in the history of their discursive construction. Similarly, in this chapter I examine the discursive, social, economic, and political conditions that create mental illness in China and its cultural and historical specificity. The Chinese folk saying *qiong feng le* means "poverty causes madness." As is the case elsewhere, mental illnesses in China are culturally specific (Kleinman 1980). They are not just about mind and body, but also about external power structures and inequalities based on gender, class, and ethnicity. With this chapter I look at one case study of socially induced mental illness in China: depression and suicide among bureaucratic officials and the ways these particular distresses shape the construction of personhood.

## PSYCHOLOGICAL AND PSYCHIATRIC DISORDERS

According to existing research and the counselors and psychiatrists I spoke with, people with *xinli wenti* (psychological issues) may suffer subhealth (see Introduction) but still be considered basically "healthy." At a voluntary informational session at MKH in the summer of 2012, one of the chief psychiatrists, Dr. Mi (MKH-2012-d2), talked about change in people's attitudes toward psychological issues and the differences between psychological issues and psychiatric diseases (*jingshen jibing*). Dr. Mi stated that in the early days of counseling (early 1980s), those who called the clinic would tell the operator that they were consulting on behalf of someone else, because many then equated counseling or psychological issues with psychiatric diseases, which were stigmatized at the time. Now people more freely admit that they have psychological issues. For Dr. Mi and colleagues, psychological issues refer to situated psychological developments or personality conflicts. Such issues arise temporarily within a certain context, for example emotional instability. In general, those with psychological issues can function normally in society. However, Dr. Mi claimed that psychiatric diseases may involve brain dysfunction leading to obstacles in one's *zhi, qing, xing, yi* (cognition, emotion, behavior, and will). The sufferer cannot function properly and requires hospital treatment or a guardian's supervision. According to Dr. Mi, the key difference lies in awareness: those who suffer psychological issues are aware of their conditions, while those who suffer psychiatric issues are usually not. Everyone can develop psychological issues owing to lost love, failures in exams, or interpersonal conflicts. These issues can be modified, alleviated, or cured with the help of family, friends, or counselors. However, if not treated, psychological issues may eventually develop into psychiatric diseases with symptoms including hallucination and delusions, which often require psychopharmaceutical intervention at specialized psychiatric hospitals and possibly psychotherapeutic treatment. Like many psychiatrists in China, Dr. Mi emphasized the symptoms of psychological and psychiatric disorders and their treatment (predominantly cognitive behavioral therapy or biomedicine) rather than their (social) causes. In the following, I discuss the social, political, and economic factors contributing to mental distress in China.

## Cultural contributions to mental distress

Culture shapes experiences of suffering (Kleinman 1988). People's ways of thinking about stress, appropriate emotional responses to it, and expectations for how to act are shaped through social and cultural contexts. Chinese people's mental well-being is frequently associated with stress arising from the family environment or intergenerational relationships owing to the self's embeddedness in networks. In Chinese culture, family is perceived as *da wo* (the "great self") and an individual is embedded in the family. Confucian relationalism is based on personal duties to others and on social goals, in contrast to an emphasis within Western individualism on personal rights (Bedford and Hwang 2003). An individual in Chinese society is obligated to maintain a well-functioning family, even as, in recent times, privatization has eroded familial and communal ties, and a growing emphasis has been placed on individual autonomy or individual-centered ethics.

Guilt and shame are common manifestations of psychological distress and are often considered symptoms of mental disorder (Hsiao et al. 2006). The subjective experience of guilt emerges when one feels that one has violated a moral order and is responsible for a negative outcome. In recent years in China, EAP counselors have found that the pressure and stress experienced by employees in big corporations do not really come from work *per se*, but rather from guilt over failure to develop appropriate relationships with their children and failure to fulfill filial piety (Fu 2016) owing to the demands of neoliberal socioeconomic conditions.

Because interpersonal dynamics are central to the Chinese concept of the self and the way the self is constructed, negotiated, and regulated (Kipnis 2012), deviations in interpersonal dynamics are relevant to the experience of distress and may contribute to perceptions of psychopathology. Consonant with the influence of Confucian philosophy, "face" is a collective concept. "Loss of face" not only involves an individual, but also families and ancestors (King and Bond 1985). Fei-Hsui Hsiao and colleagues (2006) illustrate that Chinese people's negative perceptions of themselves or loss of face as a result of transgressed personal identity and family reputation lead them to feel guilt, shame, disappointment, and hopelessness. Michael Phillips and Veronica Pearson (1996) argue that by emphasizing the family as central to the management of life's problems, Confucian values influence Chinese people to experience weak family support as psychologically distressing and to feel shame when they cannot live up to expectations for giving such support. Family conflict is frequently associated with depression among Chinese people (Zhang et al. 1997). Hsiao and colleagues (2006) thus suggest that therapies such as Western psychotherapy that emphasize patients' autonomy may be culturally inappropriate because they fail to recognize the Chinese mode of embedding the self in social relationships and the cultural expectations for appropriate roles.

In Chinese society, *zuo ren* (to be a person) is to put oneself in a social network and conform to interpersonal cultural standards. A network constitutes a satisfactory level of psychological and interpersonal equilibrium (Hsu 1971) that is key to health (Hong 2016). To maintain health, one needs to pay attention to self-care, self-education, and self-liberation as well as eight (moral) "drugs," namely, affection, kindness, integrity, tolerance, filial piety, genuineness, devotion, and the expectation that one will not be rewarded (Hong 2016). In this way, Hong Zhaoguang (2016) integrates self-care with relational care, which dovetails with the idea of a network as part of the self. Compassion and love for others maintains a harmonious family life and interpersonal relationships, which are crucial for health and longevity. All these factors for healthy living in fact resonate with the goals of the government's political project of a harmonious society. However, while the recent discourse on health emphasizes individual efforts, self-cultivation, and interpersonal relationships, broader sociopolitical processes, including China's economic transformations, the increasing privatization of health care, and the reduced public support for health since the mid-1990s, are too often ignored.

## Political definition of mental distress

It might be helpful to think of the relation of the Chinese state to mental distress in terms of previous attempts to control the population. In Mao's era, millions of Chinese were mobilized to participate in various political campaigns. The goal was to reconfigure society and reinvigorate the population for unity and socialist construction. Today, a similar mobilization is underway, if far less formal or explicit. To sustain sociopolitical stability and "care" for the people in China, the government promotes, both directly and indirectly, lay diagnosis – that is, people's surveillance of their own mental health and the mental well-being of their loved ones and those surrounding them. This new, informal and de-professionalized mass movement assists the government in balancing political control and treatment of mental health issues. However, it can be detrimental to both those who are "diagnosed" and those who really suffer mental distress.

Recently, claiming to care for those who are mentally ill, the Bureau of Public Health and Family Planning in the Shuangliu District of Chengdou, Sichuan Province, made an announcement via the microblog Weibo encouraging the public to identify those who behave "abnormally" or who conform to a set of criteria (Zha 2016). The reward for "diagnosing" one case of mental illness is RMB 350 (US$50.00), which some Internet users ridiculed as a new money-making opportunity. The eleven criteria for "mental illness" include that those under scrutiny have been: (1) once admitted to a mental hospital and are currently at home; (2) chained up or locked in at home because of a mental disorder; (3) frequently saying something that others cannot understand or that does not conform to social reality (e.g., talking with gods); (4) frequently quarrelling with others, beating people up, throwing or breaking things without reason; (5) frequently talking to themselves with a crazed or blank expression; (6) behaving in public eccentrically, wearing untidy clothing or nothing at all; (7) being overly suspicious, suspecting that everyone is gossiping about them or plotting to harm them; (8) being overactive, running around erratically, or interfering with matters irrelevant to them; (9) acting in an overly quiet, indifferent, or cold manner, doing nothing but lying in bed; (10) attempting suicide or harming themselves; (11) refusing to go outside (for school, work, or social interacton). After receiving much criticism from the public, the district admitted that these were only early symptoms of mental disorders and were not actually diagnostic criteria; however, they remain as publicly known principles for recognizing mental illness.

This is not the first time that the masses have been mobilized to identify and "diagnose" mental illness (see Zha 2016). If such informal mental illness diagnosis is manipulated within the classified *dang'an* (personal dossier) system (see Yang 2011a), the effect can be devastating. On December 3, 2002, Tang Guoji, a well-known writer in China's Hunan Province, received an unexpected phone call asking him to go to the township government to deal with procedures regarding his "mental disability." Tang was shocked: this was the first time he had heard that he had been officially identified as "mentally ill." He had experienced many personal misfortunes and unfair treatment over the previous 20 years that had, to that point, been incomprehensible to him. It now became clear that they were related to his *dang'an*. Tang graduated from Hunan Yiyang Teachers' College in 1983. Yet, even during years when teachers were in high demand, he was unable to find a teaching job. While a well-known writer, he could only find work at the canteen of a township middle school in Yiyang, Hunan Province. In his forties, he was not able to find himself a marriage partner. The informal diagnosis, the so-called *zuzhi yijian* (institutional opinions), based on the subjective evaluation of one of his teachers at Hunan Yiyang Teachers' College, had been filed in his *dang'an*, ruined his career, and damaged his life. As a student, Tang had actively taken part in a petition to change the teachers' education process and his "diagnosis" seemed to be a retaliation (see Chapter 2 on "petitioning bigotry").

The "diagnosis" of mental illness by non-medical experts (e.g., politicians or government agencies) has been used to serve diverse purposes ranging from retaliating against petitioners to scrutinizing and pathologizing people in order to obtain government support for mental illness, all of which further intensifies the stigma attached to mental illness and results in discrimination against those who actually do suffer mental distress in China (see Chapter 4 on stigma).

FROM SOMATIZATION TO THE EMPHASIS ON
PSYCHOLOGICAL AND EMOTIONAL HEALTH

Today, people express mental health concerns both somatically and psychologically, rather than exclusively somatically, as often was the case prior to, during, and after the Cultural Revolution. Arthur Kleinman (1980, 1986) examines the prevailing neurasthenia in China as a possible "somatization" of depression in the aftermath of that tumultuous period. Even though somatization rests on a conceptual divide between the somatic and the psychological, Kleinman explores the social conditions that encouraged the somatic articulation of distresses. Other lines of inquiry about somatic complaints deriving from possible psychological or psychiatric disorders address the cultural habitus of undifferentiating body from mind in Chinese medical contexts (Ots 1994; Zhang 2007). Further, in studying Chinese body culture through sports, Susan Brownell (1995) examines how social tensions are routinely expressed in bodily metaphors, which may explain from a different perspective why the Chinese often use bodily symptoms or somatic complaints to describe their distress, whether originally mental, emotional, or physical. That is, societal pressure could force individuals to express their distress somatically if they have control over their illness at some level.

Brownell suggests that Chinese people are caught in a web of interdependencies, the most acute of which link the individual, the family, and the state. Such interdependencies and their points of conflict are expressed in conceptions about the body and its physiology. Brownell contends that somatization has characterized Chinese culture since ancient times; despite changes, the web of dependencies remains nearly inescapable to this day. As a result, one should recognize that the boundaries between the body, the family, and the state are more fluid in China than in the West. Individual bodies in China are conceptualized as interlinked, the boundaries between bodies as permeable

(Brownell 1995). An individual's body is not entirely his or her own, but is subject to demands and pressures from the state, family, or community that challenge individual autonomy. As mentioned, the self in China is fluid and embedded in social networks. The interlinking of the self and body, and the porous relationship of these aspects of the person with family and the state, are not only useful for understanding the social and political nature of mental distress, but also helpful in understanding somatization and the embodied, holistic approach to mental problems adopted by Chinese psychologists. Such holism, however, has dovetailed with the trend towards psychologization in China today, the power to broaden governmentality to intrude into people's lives more thoroughly than is typically possible in Western states founded on privacy and individual rights and supporting psyche-based psychotherapy.

*The emphasis on emotions in mental health*

With the introduction of the market economy and the incursion of Western psychology into Chinese knowledge and practice, recent discourse on public health in China has come to highlight the significance of *qingxu* (emotions) or emotional health in one's overall health. It is reported that over 70 percent of diseases (over 200 types of disease) are related to emotions (Hao 2014). Whether positive or negative, excessive emotions are considered to be the cause of illness and social disharmony (Larre and Rochat de la Vallee 1996).

By placing greater emphasis on one's emotions, one can improve psychological health, according to this view. Such a turn to emotion not only is an inward turn, deflecting people's attention away from broader socioeconomic processes, but also serves various other socio-political purposes. For instance, the promotion of happiness facilitates the manifestation of the "harmonious society" and enhances productivity and market competition to advance economic development (J. Yang

2013, 2014). Moreover, certain emotions have moralizing effects that again support the social harmony project. One example is current thinking on the idea of loneliness. Zhou Guoping (2016) distinguishes true *gudu* (loneliness) from *gudan* (aloneness) and from *wuliao* (boredom) by offering a moral orientation. While *gudan* refers to one who is impervious to interpersonal care or warmth and *wuliao* points to an empty soul who cannot be entertained, true *gudu* or loneliness, Zhou contends, is about a soul who strives to be understood by others, but is not. It is tragic.[1] *Gudu* is viewed as both "poison" and "medicine." In loneliness, if one does not complain or quit but continues to strive forward, by single mindedness one will achieve what others cannot (Zhou 2016). In this sense the emotional state is a "medicine" for accomplishment supporting the state's interests in productivity, but it may simultaneously be a "poison" isolating the self.

The sad connotations of *gudu* may also overcome people's anger and tendencies to complain, thereby stabilizing the individual and society. Yanhua Zhang (2007: 72) takes this focus further to show how treating emotions with emotions is a time-honored Chinese practice, with one emotion serving to overcome another. Within this cultural system, sadness is known to overcome anger, a stigmatized emotion. So when a person is excessively angry, bringing out sadness in their reactions may lessen their anger and thereby reduce dangerous, anti-social anger-related symptoms, but such therapies may fail to resolve the source of anger and thereby permit its recurrence. These categorizations and distinctions offer a language and conceptual framework for people to label and thereby more effectively attend to their emotional changes and inner lives, which compels them to be more self-reflexive and psychologically conscious. These discourses on emotions such as loneliness emphasize the individual as a source of his or her own distress as well as a source of his or her own improvement. Implicitly this notion of *gudu* and the reliance on the self mask the alienation caused by widespread socioeconomic dislocation as a result of China's economic restructuring. To some extent, this nuanced categorization of emotions resonates with Fred Myers's (1979) analysis of regulatory emotions that some communities place on the person as a "control feeling," to teach individuals what to feel and what not to feel, what kind of self to be and not be. In this sense, distinctions between emotions at a micro (psychological) level often get confused with emotions triggered by structural or cultural forces.

It is thus important to ask whether the current emphasis on emotions and the prevalence of discourse on emotional and psychological problems in China are an indication that psychological problems are truly intensifying, or whether they reflect growing social and governmental concerns that deserve to be addressed in order to maintain sociopolitical stability. Given widespread socioeconomic dislocation and the growing therapeutic mode of governance, which together have brought about new awareness and interpretations of social and mental distress as well as the need to treat them, the answer may be both. Within these trends it is vital not to let the focus on individual responsibilities overshadow the role of the state in the expansion of the negative emotional effects associated with widening economic gaps resulting from social and market reforms. As mentioned, the nuanced distinction of different notions of individual feelings of being alone or loneliness obscures the kind of alienation caused by state-led privatization and economic restructuring. Indeed, in China, sustaining social stability is seen as just as important as, if not more important than, developing the market economy, which requires realigning emotional cultures, "making the economic self and emotions more closely harnessed to instrumental actions" (Illouz 2007: 23). Emotions such as happiness have been constructed as therapeutic and influential in promoting productivity in China (Yang 2013), while the containment and pathologization of anger and discontentment has been highlighted to manage mass unemployment and sustain social stability (Yang 2016).

Scholars of China (Yan 1996; Kipnis 1997) have studied emotion as it arises both to support and to subvert bureaucratic power in China in terms of *renqing* (human feeling: empathy or compassion) and *guanxi* (social ties). By contrasting the privileged status of emotion in Western societies with the Chinese devaluation of emotion as a social force, Sulamith Potter (1988) believes that while the Chinese have a rich emotional life, they do not ground social order in the emotional life of individuals. However, critiquing Potter's reductive description of the role of emotion in Chinese society, Haiyan Lee (2007: 3) notes the multivalent, heterogeneous, and extensive discourses of sentiment related in a wide array of texts devoted to the subjects of love, feeling, desire, and sympathy, particularly since the late Qing dynasty. Lee examines the signification of emotion as the legitimizing basis for a new social order or for the reconceptualization of identity and sociality in emotive terms as a fundamental transformation of modernity.

The increasing importance of emotions in China reveals the seeming rise of individual-centered ethics (Lee 2011; Yan 2011; Kipnis 2012) and the penetration of therapeutic techniques and languages into a growing number of social domains. Lisa Rofel (2007: 6) claims that "the desiring self" is evident in consumerism, labor, and sexual choices, shifting China away from the collective consciousness of the socialist era to novel meanings of modernity. Under these conditions, people have greater opportunities to seek satisfaction for immediate personal needs and explore their inner emotional world. Meanwhile, new forms of emotional management have become gradually embedded in China's process of "modernization" (Hanser 2008). "Emotion-work" propagated through the advice industry fuels individual reflexivity in more private spheres, such as parenthood (Kuan 2015). The boom of "inner child" emotion pedagogies in contemporary China represents a convergence of events and sociohistorical circumstances that has brought adapted versions of psychotherapeutic and New Age spiritual discourse to China, creating both a distillation and an expansion of Western psychotherapeutic ideologies of language, emotion, and self (Pritzker 2016). The emphasis on individual emotions in various social domains in China has not only facilitated the construction of an emotional self that banks on emotions as avenues for knowledge production, self-governance, and self-formation; it also constitutes emotive worlds with "cultural meanings and social relationships that are very compressed together," and this compact compression confers on emotions their energetic and semiconscious character (Illouz 2007: 3). Indeed, emotions derive their power from the fact that they are a deeply internalized and unrefined aspect of action, not because they are insufficiently socioculturally informed, but because they are excessively so (Illouz 2007: 3). Further, emotions go beyond the dichotomy of cognition and bodily sensation by including both of them (see Ahmed 2004).

*Anxiety: an epochal syndrome of the rapidly changing Chinese society*

Scholars of China also trace the historical, cultural, and social constructions of emotional and psychological disorders, including anxiety. While Chinese psychologists treat moderate anxiety as an individual adaptive response anticipating potential risks or pain and pathologize excessive anxiety, Chinese sociologist Zhou Xiaohong (2014) contends that anxiety in China, understood broadly, is a social symptom of the changing society and shifting political economy. Zhou traces its origins to the late nineteenth century.

Zhou (2014) argues that while China has made remarkable achievements in the past 30 years, many Chinese still believe that both social development and the improvement of their personal lives are too slow. This belief, together with the pressure of a competitive milieu in which people wish to become more preeminent than their peers and fear lagging behind, has gradually evolved into a widespread "national anxiety." This national anxiety contrasts starkly with the national character described by Lin Yutang (1994: 76), who, in the 1930s and

1940s, characterized the Chinese populace as experiencing widespread "contentment," "leisure," and a "carefree" life. In a society that changes relatively slowly, the prevailing social attitude is often an acceptance of fate, contentment, or passivity.[2] But the widespread anxiety the Chinese are experiencing today is, at least partly, a sociopsychological reaction to rapid social changes.

Zhou (2014) further contends that reforms that began in 1978 completely changed Chinese society, but, in the end, national anxiety grew deeper and more widespread, and eventually became an epochal syndrome, for several reasons. First, the implementation of a market economy greatly changed Chinese society, giving rise to the current "GDP worship." The higher the respect for GDP growth, the slower the Chinese feel change is taking place and the more restless and anxious people have become. Second, because of the rapid social transformations, the original social order has been challenged. In the words of Chinese anthropologist Fei Xiaotong (1999: 316), this has brought about a "more pressing crisis in the psychological order." Unfamiliarity and uncertainty caused by change have led to social anxiety; people now feel "at a loss" about what course to take. Third, the market economy has stimulated money worship, which, combined with the national anxiety over being "left behind," has resulted in an experience of individual restlessness. Fei (1999: 315) suggests that Chinese society will eventually establish a social mentality within which "each individual can live peacefully and freely," but current sociopolitical-economic conditions do not support this.

## SOCIAL, ECONOMIC, AND POLITICAL FACTORS ASSOCIATED WITH MENTAL DISTRESS: "OFFICIALS' HEARTACHE"

In China, the public often call depression *qingsu ganmao* (emotional cold), or *xinling ganmao* (the cold of the soul). Besides a heart-emotion, depression has also been deemed *lanse bingdu* (blue virus), involving not only psychological or emotional dysfunction but also brain dysfunction. Depression is China's second most commonly diagnosed disease causing death (exceeded only by heart disease). Depression-related deaths such as suicides exceed traffic fatalities. According to some estimates, more than 260 million people struggled with at least mild depression in 2011 (Zhang 2017). In 2007, China's Medical Association estimated that two-thirds of depression sufferers had harbored suicidal thoughts at least once, and 15 percent to 25 percent ended their own lives (Zhang 2017).[3]

Factors contributing to depression as a disease of brain dysfunction are complicated, but most of my informants – grassroots officials – can name specific social factors, for example pressure at work that exhausted them so much that they became overwhelmed and eventually depressed. They argue that if these conditions were improved, their depression might well lighten. Xu Kaiwen (2016) uses *shu lilun* or "tree theory" to explain the social factors associated with depression and suicide. This theory has three main components: first, "the roots of the tree," the family environment in which one grows up; second, "tree trunks," one's social support system as well as one's beliefs, ideals, and values; and, third, "tree leaves," one's sense of achievement and self-affirmation. In general, for Xu, suicides in China are attributed to social processes. Suicide of university students, according to him, is predominantly derived from family issues surrounding education. For grassroots officials, depression and suicide are mainly attributed to the work environment, the autocratic bureaucratic culture. Xu's theory speaks to how Chinese psy experts capture the intricate ties between people and their mental distress and how the biomedical views of depression or suicide add little understanding to accounts of well-being in China. Many scholars argue that suicide in the Chinese context is not primarily caused by mental distress (Pearson and Liu 2002) but entails social and political factors, for example family power struggles (Wu 2010).

While many in China may associate depression with celebrities like Cui Yongyuan, Zhang Guorong, and San Mao, or members of the middle class, the highest rate of depression is actually found among members of underprivileged groups, especially those who have been laid off from state enterprises and those who are left behind in the countryside. The rate of depression among those who received social aid or poverty relief is three times the general rate of depression in China (Zhang Jin 2014). Poverty can cause depression; depression impoverishes people even more – a vicious cycle.

Alex Neitzke (2016) suggests that depression be best understood in terms of systems of power and oppression in which an individual is situated. For grassroots Chinese officials, depression offers a way for us to understand their social world. To some extent, depression is an "illness of power," but not only are they rendered "victims" of the power hierarchy in an autocratic bureaucracy, they themselves are also part and parcel of that system of power, exacerbating their distress. Some bureaucrats I interviewed engaged in corruption and became distressed because of their insecurity and uncertainty about their prospects, and because of their awareness of how twisted and corrupt the system is in which they find themselves with no way to behave according to their more traditional values.

Since the neurobiologization of depression in the 1990s, depression has been used to interrogate workers' subjectivities (Rose and Abi-Rached 2013). This neurobiological turn highlights the connection of depression to economic rationality and degenders what was formerly an "illness of emotion" (mainly affecting women) to an "illness of inaction" (Ehrenberg 2010). Depression not only disrupts overall well-being, but from the state's perspective also interferes with worker productivity, leading to high direct medical costs and indirect economic costs associated with this mental illness.

The suicide rate among Chinese officials has recently been on the rise.[4] These deaths share common features. Most occur among men between 40 and 60.[5] The cause of suicide is usually rapidly identified by employers and investigators as a set of medical and psychological conditions: *qi benren yali guo da* (personally experienced excessive pressure), *jingshen fudan guozhong* (exceptional stress), *jiaolv* (anxiety), or, most predominantly, *yiyu zheng* (depression).[6] The official reports sometimes include brief interviews with colleagues or family members, revealing personal details about the deceased such as their suffering from "insomnia," "a bad mood," or "low spirits," and highlighting these deaths as resulting from private, psychological issues. However, employers and government investigators diagnose these individuals with depression, anxiety, or other psychological disorders after death and without recourse to medical experts. The presence of psychotropic drugs like estazolam and oryzanol in the offices or cars of the deceased seems to corroborate the informal diagnoses (Fang et al. 2011). These drugs are nevertheless prescribed for a variety of conditions in China, not just depression. These reports invariably describe these officials as dedicated public servants with promising political prospects who were, unfortunately, susceptible to psychological dysfunctions (e.g., uncontrollable impulses), a characterization that serves to homogenize them and to advance a linear relationship between stress, depression, and suicide. Such homogenization and pathologization delegitimize the deceased as rational political actors and implicitly promote an ideal opposite: a subject who is rational, masterful, and psychologically healthy. In general, these media reports describe public servants collectively as a group at high risk for suicide, and they recommend that more psychotherapeutic services be made available to them (Fang et al. 2011).

Increasing openness in China to a biomedical idea of mental illness has resulted in greater acceptance of depression as biomedical, rather than an ideological (as in Mao's era) or a socially induced problem. The famous former CCTV anchor Cui Yongyuan blogged in 2012, "Damn, the frequent association of depression with corrupt officials has ruined the good reputation of this disease [its biomedical definition]." Linking to his 2005 public confession of his personal suffering from depression, which drove home the message that depression is a real disease requiring biomedical treatment and doctor's care, his blogging highlights the politicization of depression in China, a process in which it is represented in public discourse as an impediment to work rather than a hazard of work in the public sector.

While historically, in Chinese culture, an emphasis on interpersonal harmony has been at the core of one's personhood (see Hsu 1971), the media's representation of biomedical depression as the main cause of officials' suicides is widely viewed as necessary for the ubiquitous post-2004 political project of constructing a "harmonious society." Individuals who cannot make it need to be sacrificed for the greater collective good of those who can manage in this new economy.

However, my ethnographic research shows that the prevalence of *qian guize* (hidden rules) in Chinese bureaucracy is the main factor contributing to officials' "heartache," including anxiety, depression, and suicide (see also He 2011). Similarly, a 2009 survey conducted by *Renmin Luntan*, an offshoot of *People's Daily*, on officials' work pressure also showed that of 5,800 officials surveyed, 64.65 percent believed that the pressure felt by officials is mainly due to the impact of *qian guize* on their political prospects. Mid-ranking cadres report the worst mental health conditions, and officials between the ages of 30 and 50 tend to report the most stress because of pressure for promotion in a competitive environment where merit is determined by *qian guize* (Fang et al. 2011; Liu 2014).[7]

Coined by Chinese journalist-turned-historian Wu Si (2001), *qian guize* are hidden rules that shadow, complement, bypass, or twist the operation of formal, established rules in Chinese institutions. They are informal codes of behavior that range from prescriptions for proper demeanor to minor rule-bending to more serious transgressions aimed at amassing wealth or benefits, including nepotism, flattery, and bribery. These are interest-based strategies defining access to resources, including career advancement and pay raises.

*Qian guize* underpin what amounts to an autocracy – the idiosyncratic rule of individuals rather than the predictable rule of law. It is hard to pinpoint what exactly *qian guize* are in any specific context. Most of my informants indicated that navigating *qian guize* of the bureaucracy requires *tihui* (embodied understanding), meaning they must read fluctuating meanings of body language, a look, a wink, or a pat on one's shoulder, depending on context. Failure to understand *qian guize* leads to consequences. In the words of one official in charge of the road system in Zhangqiu: "You have to interpret [the implicit messages of superiors] accurately and speak accordingly. Every day you walk on thin ice; if [you are] not careful you will fall into deep waters…. No matter how healthy you are, you will sooner or later become *depressed*; it's so important to twist yourself to fit the system."

Many of my informants stated outright that they must perform as *shuangmian ren* (two-faced people) to survive; they claim to serve "the people" through their work, but they must attend to their own personal interests because of the demands of *qian guize*. Many ended up in what Gregory Bateson (1973) deems "double binds": social relationships that require permanent management of contradictions. The double bind imposes irreconcilable (ethical) demands on the subject in situations in which he or she has no meaningful way to respond or escape. Double binds can produce anger that endangers social harmony and so is often subconsciously contained, giving rise to inner rage that is channeled unconsciously or indirectly into everyday speech and acts.

In addition to a work environment governed by hidden rules and contradictions, officials' distress may also relate to the severity of current anticorruption measures. Officials accused of corruption may be penalized through *shuanggui* – dual designation of time and location for interrogation – an extralegal procedure overseen by the Party's disciplinary committees to detain and interrogate them (Sapio 2008; Chu 2011). Psychological manipulation and physical torture, including sleep deprivation, simulated drowning, and beating, are reportedly common during *shuanggui*. To avoid this scenario, conceal corruption, and avoid prosecution, some officials choose to end their lives; according to Chinese law, death ends the corruption investigation. These deaths are then reported as due to "depression." Commentators have even wondered whether President Xi's anticorruption campaign, which ramped up dramatically starting in 2012, may purposefully *sha ji jing hou* (kill the chicken to frighten the monkey), punishing some as a warning to others. The campaign probably exacerbates the pressure officials experience and may directly push them to suicide.

## CONCLUSION

In this chapter I have discussed the Chinese concepts of mental health and mental illness and the social, economic, and political contributions to mental distress that have created new frameworks for understanding mental instabilities in China. I have also explored how Chinese cultural history impacts forms of distress and their manifestations. Since mental distress in China is attributed more to external forces than to biology, I have analyzed symptoms of mental illness that demonstrate this external influence on distress ("officials' heartache").

I have also examined contemporary psychological practices in order to understand both insights and limitations of psychological approaches to Chinese selfhood. Psychological practice may recognize that in China the self and even the body are fundamentally relational, existing in a social network. Distress may be understood with this awareness in mind. Local psy experts are, at times, used by the state to construct client subjectivities that are identified with state interests and to use the repair of distress for social control. In this process, counselors may actually demonstrate an understanding of the relational selfhood and body that exists in China, and claim to adopt an embodied and holistic approach to mental distress.

However, more often than not, counselors end up emphasizing the inner self and individual responsibility for resolving personal difficulties and suffering. Paradoxically, while mental illnesses are mainly associated with socioeconomic processes, the psychological toolkits offered by psy experts for maintaining psychological health are mainly biomedical and personal. In general psychological practices today in China tend to focus on personal solutions and attitude adjustments to alleviate distress. This approach fails to confront the power of the state, which itself is entwined with psychology and emotion, as it attempts to govern its population through a period of rapid social change. I have introduced three oppositions that are interconnected. The first is Western practices and knowledge versus Chinese holistic understandings and treatments. The second is the responsibility for distress that falls to the state and social change versus individual mental weaknesses or situated reactions. The third is situated versus biological impetuses to mental suffering.

Chinese writer and counselor Bi Shumin (2012), in her book entitled *No Man is an Island*, offers *guanxi* (social ties) as a type of "medicine" for depression and mental distress. Bi observes that everyone is embedded within social networks and all human activities can be categorized into three kinds of relationships: each human being's relationship with themselves, with other people, and with nature. Bi contends that all those who suffer depression have problems with *guanxi*. That is, conflicted *guanxi* contributes to depression. However, while Bi's observations may entail implicit criticism of the state-sponsored promotion of individual-centered ethics and the emphasis on individual autonomy in some schools of psychotherapy in China, she augments these accounts only by pointing to interpersonal relationships among autonomous beings. She emphasizes *guanxi* decoupled from socioeconomic structures, for example by highlighting faults in one's orientation to others – misunderstandings, betrayals, quarreling, cheating, or contempt – rather than offering a more penetrating critique of the alienating effects of widespread socioeconomic dislocation that have resulted from state-led economic restructuring since the mid-1990s. Bi's ideas represent some of the tensions in psychological thinking and practices in China. They capture the possibilities and limits of contemporary Chinese psychological practice. There is an acknowledgement – or at least an instinct – that using primarily Western tools or state-recommended notions of individual responsibility to help people in distress will not work in China. But there is an unwillingness to go the extra step of criticizing imported ideas and the state's adapted focus on individuals. The unwillingness to go beyond the limits of shallow critiques of biological interventions and individualism may be due to the insidious power and hegemony of China's reductive and homogenizing therapeutic governance.

The Chinese state develops therapeutic techniques that are equally as ineffective as borrowed Western approaches – such as the condemnation of suicide victims as inadequate to the social and economic demands of the times by labeling them as "depressed." These state-governed techniques of condemnation may be influenced by Western emphases on the individual, but they are transformed in the Chinese application. Indeed, it is not simple Western tools that are at issue, but Chinese manipulation and incorporation of those tools into their own sociopolitical-economic goals. For example, the Chinese approach to mental distress considers social factors, but centers them predominantly on the family and interpersonal relationships without contextualizing these relationships in broader social, economic, and political processes. This approach will be further demonstrated in Chapter 2 in my discussion of new mental "illnesses," which mainly result from China's recent economic restructuring.

# 2 | New Chinese Mental "Illnesses"

Depression is the cause of all suicides committed by officials; mental illness
afflicts all those who petition [against the state].

*A Chinese folk saying*

"Internet addiction" itself is a false concept.

*Tang Yinghong, 2016*

The Chinese media frequently report on new psychological conditions. Although media outlets and experts link these conditions with the ubiquitous stress associated with socioeconomic transformation, the focus is often on individual psychological illness. In a recent TV news report, for example, one family described how their son had become addicted to video games. The report included corroboration from a psychologist who said the child would require residential treatment for the addiction that, in his view, had taken hold of his brain. The parents both worked long hours, and the son was nearly ready to sit upper-level exams in his high school. The report focused on the devastation caused by the child's video gaming, but it indicated little about the stress of student exams or the intense competition within China's utilitarian, grade-oriented educational system. Nor did it discuss the context in which video games have become integral to Chinese consumer culture, or the reasons why both parents in the family might need to work overtime. This suggests that, alongside the real pain of new, imputed "mental illnesses" like "video-game addiction" or "Internet addiction," there might be more to understand.

In this chapter I analyze a set of what have been identified as new mental diseases – including *xialibaren zhenghou qun* (country bumpkin syndrome), *gongzhu bing* (princess disease), *wumai yiyuzheng* (smog depression/blues), *shangfang cheng yin* or *shangfang pian zhi* (petitioning addiction, petitioning bigotry, or litigious disease), *shiye zonghezheng* (unemployment complex syndrome), *kongxin bing* (empty-heart disease), and *wangyin* (Internet addiction). These "diseases" have been created in the past decade by the Chinese media and the medical and psychiatric community and reiterated by the general public. Drawing on theory regarding the social and cultural construction of mental illness (Foucault 1976), the contested boundaries between mental illness and social "deviance" or social differences (Busfield 1989, 2012), and idioms of distress (Nichter 2010), I examine how these new disorders psychologize or medicalize "deviance," and how some of the diagnoses depend on stereotypical conceptions of identity, as opposed to embracing differences. My analysis focuses on the way social, moral, economic, and political issues are psychologized and thus downplayed through these new "diseases," as well as on the uniquely Chinese characteristics of this psychologization process.

## ILLNESSES AND IDIOMS OF DISTRESS

Since the mid-1990s, psychologization of distress of all kinds has been pervasive in China (J. Yang 2015). Psychological self-help literature and biographical confessional talk shows are popular, while discourses of mood, affect, and emotion have spread, particularly in big cities. Media and Internet sites trade widely in psychological jargon, now well represented in public parlance (see Feng 1996; J. Yang 2015).

Concurrent with this widespread public discourse, new medical diagnoses of psychological disorders have multiplied. For example, eating disorders had previously not been considered illnesses in China, but with recent translations into Chinese (see Lee 1991), *yanshizheng* or "eating disorders" have become new diseases with a rapid increase in cases. An unprecedented number of Chinese now have a diagnosed mental illness (see Introduction). In part, this has resulted from new definitions of mental illness and new procedures for psychiatric diagnosis. For example, while many more people are diagnosed with depression, Sing Lee (2011) points out that until a few years ago it took three months to diagnose a case of depression; now it takes two weeks for diagnosis and administration of a drug. But shifts in diagnostic procedures alone do not explain the dramatic increase in kinds and incidences of mental illness. As has long been argued, illness is both a somatic experience and a social construct. Foucault (1976) showed how psychological conditions developed in step with the status of psychology and psychologists. Others have studied the power of the medical profession and political structures in defining illness (Laing 1961).

Still others consider illness a socially conditioned response to stress. Richard Cloward and Frances Piven (1979) argue that the way people respond to stress is socially constructed. These responses are channeled by the normative rules of society; they are socially regulated. To understand "deviant" behaviors and feelings – say, playing 10 straight hours of video games – we need to understand the cognitive, moral, and bodily frameworks through which people process stress: for example, the stress of a test-based education system.

Mark Nichter (2010) uses the term "idiom of distress" to capture a similar idea. For Nichter, proliferating illnesses are actually cultural "syndromes." He suggests that expressions of distress may be drawn from a number of culturally and personally available meaning complexes. Idioms of distress provide a promising venue for exploring common distress and moral confusion. For example, the new Chinese category of *gongzhu bing* (princess disease) refers to a kind of (young) Chinese woman who insists on being treated like a princess, someone who overspends and pampers herself, living a luxurious lifestyle. These girls are seen as over-confident to the point of deviancy, and their clothes, attitudes, and manners mimic what they imagine are those of a real princess. Cloward and Piven (1979) might argue that to understand these behaviors, we need to understand the stressors that affect the girls. In this case, a generation of young people, the product of China's one-child policy, who have lived through the recent transformation of the Chinese economy, face conflicting expectations from their parents, who might want their children to reflect their ascending economic status, but who also place significant traditional expectations on their offspring. With the shifting gender ideology that values hyper-femininity in the reform era and the politicized re-traditionalization of China (see Yu 2006), many girls are expected to both succeed in the world of work and fulfill traditional gender roles. Behaving like a princess reflects some of these stresses. Nichter (2010) would argue that we can only understand princess disease in terms of the broader culture in China, which has been turning away from social support toward valuing individual consumption – a princess is one "idiom" in which cultural and mental distress is expressed.

Nichter cautions against using such interpretations to deem illnesses less serious or genuine than diseases attributed to biological causes. Rather, he suggests that ethnographic accounts of cultural variation in illness have often ignored the pragmatics of expressing social or political ills through somatization (though see Kleinman 1986). While the notion of cultural influence on physical symptoms unexplained by biology is not new (e.g., Townsend and Carbone 1980), the concept of idioms of distress provides an expanded and more nuanced understanding of how non-biological, extra-corporeal distress emerges in the form of bodily ill-being. Similarly, Nichter and Thompson (2006) illustrate with empirical research how North Americans use dietary supplements both as self-governance and as an idiom of distress or concern for self and others. Other anthropological work has contributed to understanding the relationship between distress and medicalization, on the one hand, and sociopolitical issues, on the other (Yarris 2014).

## PATHOLOGIZING DEVIANT BEHAVIORS, EXPERIENCES, AND POPULAR SOCIAL ATTITUDES

Adopting medical terms transforms a variety of social, moral, and psychological phenomena into new "illnesses." *Xialibaren zhenghouqun* (country bumpkin syndrome) first appeared around the mid-1990s and refers to newly rich Chinese who overconsume and display luxury goods, while living a life that, in other ways, closely resembles that of a stereotypical, unsophisticated rural person. The syndrome captures the contradiction between what one aspires for in one's heart and what one lives out, between one's aspiration for something elegant and distinct, and one's actual practice, manifesting the tastes or lifestyles of common folk. Commentators contend that those who prefer to present themselves as people who can afford high culture and enjoy showing off their good taste by consuming high-end commodities construct a *chao wo* (super self), while the activities they typically engage in remain more mundane and derive from their habitual rustic ways of life, revealing their *ben wo* (true self). This divided subjectivity, which is based on stereotypical characteristics of China's new rich rather than a continuum of ways of their living, differs from the divided self conceptualized by Arthur Kleinman and his colleagues (2011).

From the perspective of idioms of distress, the illness is a particular reaction to a transitional time in China. People are facing contradictory influences from both the West and Chinese tradition. One wants to change and follow the newest trends, but at the same time one is unlikely to entirely cast off habitual practices. One's value orientation is in flux and shifting. The "syndrome" describes this popular social attitude and subjectivity that indexes the ruptures of Chinese society resulting from socioeconomic transformation (see Osburg 2013 on the contradictory practices of the new rich in China).

Another emerging social "epidemic" is called *jinqian jikezheng* (money hunger disease) (A Su 2014). In this discourse, a market-driven society is centered on profit and interest and people's rush to obtain them. The emotional reality of this setup is characterized by ecstasy when one makes money and panic when one loses it. Everything is about money; value, success, and subjectivity are entirely based on the amount of cash one can make or possess. Money has become the torch guiding people and their livelihood: poor people try hard to earn it, while the rich work to make yet more of it. That is, the more money people have, the greater their desire to increase their wealth. Ultimately, what they have is only money; many are poor deep inside. Such money hunger has a deep psychological cause: a lack of love, certainty, and security. People are seeking external value owing to this inner lack. In their hearts, what they are chasing is not money, but rather spiritual fulfillment, such as that evidenced by love, acceptance, and attention (A Su 2014). This can help explain the Chinese "epidemic" of buying. Of course, there are structural reasons for increasing consumption in China. Not only has the country become the world's largest manufacturer, but the contrast between the present surplus of consumer goods and the recent past, in which goods were scarce, is still vivid for people. In part, "country bumpkin syndrome" is an expression of the jarring shift from scarcity to plenty.

In addition to overconsumption, for many in China, hoarding is a means of expressing the same distress over the socioeconomic shifts. "Often, [people] … just buy things to fill the hollow in their hearts, and accumulating things indicates the heavy burden they carry in their minds," suggested Yamashita Hideko, a Japanese self-help writer, at a lecture in Beijing's 798 art district on November 10, 2015 (Yang Yang 2015). Hideko notes that instead of a place for relaxation, the home has become a place cluttered with an excess of useless things that people do not want to throw away. It has turned into a garbage dump. Such a situation affects one's psychological state. Hideko has become famous for her concept of *danshari*, which she developed from making her own domestic decluttering, and from yoga. It is the practice of junking unnecessary possessions and separating oneself from the drive to have and own things. By cleaning up, one gets rid of both physical and mental junk. For Hideko, the essence of *danshari* is the focus on oneself, right here, right now. Another important insight is that through disposing of superfluous things, people learn about themselves and learn how to make clear-headed decisions about career, love, and marriage.

An increasing number of Chinese people have started reviewing their surroundings at home and their mental situation in these ways, with an eye to rejecting surplus. A new type of house service is now on offer: specialists visit a client's home to provide advice on making the space neat, to find out what things clients like or dislike, and to tell them to throw away things they do not like in order to create a peaceful mind and freedom from superfluous goods. A woman who was present at Hideko's lecture shared her experience of practicing *danshari*. She said that she had suffered from depression and used to eat a lot, but was unwilling to visit a psychotherapist. After reading Hideko's book *Danshari*, she cleaned her house, ate less, lost 5 kilograms, and was on her way to recovering from depression.

With the concept of idiom of distress, it is possible to link the moralizing discourse of purity in *danshari*, which is considered a way of overcoming ill behaviors, with the excess and display of "country bumpkin syndrome." Both can be seen as reactions to distress over cultural or socioeconomic shifts. Each is structured using available cultural complexes of meaning – leading to excess or rejection. In "country bumpkin syndrome," subjects embrace what post-Mao China has to offer: more of everything, but also a link to China's recent socialist past marked by scarcity. In *danshari*, subjects can feel morally superior to those perceived as money hungry by creating a safe distance from the complex of feelings that accompany consumer goods – ironically, by paying someone to come and clear out their things. It is a way of governing one's space and one's self. However, to understand these "ill" behaviors and feelings, one must see them as a product of stress coming as much from outside as from inside the individual.

## "SMOG DEPRESSION/BLUES"

Rather than locate the source of mental distress completely within the biological body, the concept of idioms of distress allows for analysis of how the body and heart process pain coming from the outside. This richer view of mental suffering can help us understand another new "illness" emerging in China, so-called *wumai yiyuzheng*, or "smog depression/blues." Chinese economist Wang Dingding (2016) coined this term, predicting that, given the long-term heavy smog and low visibility in China's capital, smog blues will become the most frequently occurring and most widespread psychological disorder among Beijingers.

In recent years, severe air pollution has frequently engulfed China's big cities, but rather than seeing an increase in cases of respiratory system diseases, mental health experts have noted a slight increase in anxiety, neurosis, or worsening depressive symptoms among people diagnosed after exposure to polluted air. Several psychiatrists at MKH indicated that during a period of heavy smog, people often come to the hospital presenting with somatic complaints including congested chest, breathing difficulties, and constant coughing. While these physical symptoms may not be sufficiently measurable to be formally diagnosed as physical illnesses, they are considered as symptoms of psychological distress and anxiety about the possibility of developing severe illnesses owing to the bad air. Dr. Wang Jian, a psychiatrist at Beijing Huilong-guan Hospital, noted that during a "red alert," when smog is likely to remain at about 10 times the safe level of PM 2.5 for three days or longer, a large number of patients with depression and neurosis came to him and complained about their worsening symptoms after being exposed to the polluted air. Wang advises patients to stay indoors and to keep their lights on (Phillips 2015). Other psychiatrists have been more reserved about the links between smog and mental health, especially depression, as they point out that depressed patients are highly affected by all kinds of weather and environmental change – think of "winter blues" (seasonal affective disorder, SAD), known to affect people in the Northern Hemisphere. Symptoms of "winter blues" include depression, decreased energy, excessive sleeping, weight gain, a craving for carbohydrates, and so on. As a treatment, light therapy is usually advised. In China, however, the circumstances are unique. The atmospheric change here is human-driven, caused by large-scale industrial activities, often unfettered by inadequate environmental regulation, sometimes intensified by corruption. Thus, distress related to smog might have both social and environmental significance. There is also a particular incentive for the public and psy experts to pay attention to the relationship between smog and mental health, as this link could draw the attention of policy makers and compel them to deal with pollution.

A few psychiatrists I spoke with in Beijing indicated that they have encountered people coming to the hospital with typical symptoms of mild depression during a period of heavy smog, but after a trip to a fresh-air environment like Hainan Province their symptoms entirely disappeared. However, their symptoms would likely recur with another "red alert." Smog-related depression and public concerns about the health effect of pollution have partly facilitated the rapid development of eco-tourism and eco-psychology in China. For example, in suburban areas of Beijing, such as Changping, mountain-based organic farms and "heart-soul oxygen bars" have become popular tourist sites, at which psychologists counsel tourists participating in weekend excursions that are built around de-stressing activities such as shedding cornstalks and talking to animals. These eco-psychological methods regard nature as a source of meaning and therapy, and living in harmony with nature as essential to human emotional and mental well-being. This form of psychological relief combines both counseling based on traditional therapeutic modes – which rarely looks beyond the individual, family, or social dimensions of human personality – and nature-based healing to construct healthy subjects who can come to terms with the (environmental and health) effects of China's modernization and socioeconomic transformation.

### "PETITIONING ADDICTION"/"PETITIONING BIGOTRY" AND "LITIGIOUS DISEASE"

Since the mid-1990s, *baoyuan* (complaining) has been depicted in public discourse in China as a poisonous tumor and an illness. It is described as resembling bad breath: those who complain do not realize it but their interlocutors will suffer. Job counselors in Changping view complaining as an individual pathology that prevents people from getting jobs or living a fulfilled life, and even as requiring treatment. In Changping, laid-off workers who were invited to job counseling sessions organized by residents' committees would often be given hats with four Chinese characters on them: *Wo bu baoyuan* (I do not complain). One job counselor in the district viewed complaints as opposing positive psychology and remarked during a counseling session in summer 2012 that "The best mindset is to reconcile oneself to one's situation and be patient. Complaining is poisonous. It will destroy your will power, lower your status, destroy your body and mind, and reduce your enthusiasm."

Increasing disdain for complaining behaviors has consequences at all levels of Chinese society. It has now shifted the tone within one of China's long-running institutions that deals with individual grievances.

The Chinese petition system, *xinfang*, serves as an official channel for the Chinese government to handle complaints that cannot otherwise be resolved. Superior or upper-level institutions and leadership present a benevolent face to people who are wronged by local officials and deprived of the chance for a fair hearing or trial. This system claims to redress injustice and defuse unrest. Today, *xinfang* is being tested as the number of grievances increases. The term "petitioning addiction" or "petitioning bigotry" (litigious disease in other social contexts) has arisen in this context. To understand it, we first need to examine how *xinfang* operates.

According to a 2013 survey, of over 4,200 *xinfang* cases received by the Chinese government, only 558 cases (about 13 percent) were (at least partially) resolved (Yang 2013). Despite this low success rate, Chinese petitioners still believe that *xinfang* may be worth trying, especially compared to their other choices, such as going to court or "going to the streets" (protesting) (Li et al. 2012), as formally adjudicated issues in China are often decided by those with administrative power rather than those who are supposedly less subject to administrative bias (Chen 2014: 120). While *xinfang* is considered one of the most critical quasi-democratic institutions through which the Chinese government deals with resistance (Lee and Zhang 2013),[1] in reality it can take years for complainants to reach a resolution to their case.

Indeed, *xinfang* officers often perceive disgruntled petitioners as unreasonable or as making a big fuss. Recently, they have begun to consider those who habitually petition as suffering from petitioning addiction or bigotry, which resembles a notion of "litigious disease." This refers to those who putatively utilize the legal system as a vehicle to act out their fantasies and delusional preoccupations. The symptoms of litigious disease include imaginary grievances, accusations based on delusional ideation, and irrational vindictiveness toward imagined persecutors (Goldstein 1987). For people who experience real distress or grievances, *xinfang* as a culturally understandable avenue for redress is often the preferred option for attempting to reduce that distress. The increase in cases taken through the *xinfang* process makes "petitioning bigotry" an idiom of distress reflecting social and cultural stressors.

To show how the petitioning system psychiatrizes petitioners and puts them in mental hospitals as a way to control them while superficially constructing social harmony, we shall consider one example: the case of Xu Xueling from Xintai, Shandong Province (Yu 2016). About 10 years ago, Xu started to petition the central government to protest the leniency in penalizing someone from Xinwen Mining Company who seriously injured her sister. However, during her petitioning, she was "diagnosed" as "hysterical" by local petitioning officers and the government officials in charge of *wei wen* (maintaining social stability) without formal mental assessments offered by medical authorities. She was treated by the township government as one of the "unstable elements" and put in a local mental hospital, where she was forced to take medication. Xu took the drugs but vomited them out whenever possible. After her sister's case was resolved, Xu continued to petition for a *shuofa* (explanation or justice) because of her forcible medical treatment. Without diagnosis, she was sent to another mental hospital.

After she was released from that hospital, she was then accused by the local government of forcibly expropriating 37,700 yuan from the government and was sentenced to a four-year imprisonment in 2015 in the name of *xunxin zishi* (picking quarrels and provoking troubles). This time, Xu was treated independently of her "mental illness history"; she was viewed as being entirely sane, thereby fully responsible for her allegedly "forcibly expropriating money." However, Xu resisted the verdict by highlighting that she was given the money by the local government to stop her petitioning for the sake of maintaining social stability.

Xu's case demonstrates the amenability of "mental illness" to misdiagnosis and other misapplications, and its close and flexible entanglement with social and political agendas in China. We can also consider this case in relation to the concept of idioms of distress. *Xinfang*, while allowing some justice, is no longer an efficient system. It fails to cope with the rapidly escalating number of grievances and mass discontent resulting from the tumultuous transition to a market economy. China remains a one-party state that is not always accountable to its people. However, the powerful bureaucracy is threatened by private interests, and internal political struggle and competition for positions are intense. Little energy is available to meet the needs of petitioners, who, at the same time, are denigrated for a perceived weakness, *baoyuan*: for example, in the case of unemployed workers in Changping, who feel entitled to their rights and complain. Thus, petitioning addiction refers, simultaneously, to the real psychological and physical distress of petitioners (though often exacerbated by their mistreatment at the hands of *xinfang* officials), and to a social and political construct that pathologizes and even incarcerates petitioners in the name of assuring socio-political stability.

Another case highlights how the *xinfang* system tortures petitioners in ways that lead to their real mental distress and psychological suffering. In summer 2010, I met Mali, a woman in her early fifties (ZYH-2010-p2), at Dr. Wen's office at ZYH. She suffered moderate depression and anxiety; her most troubling symptom was insomnia, which really bothered her and negatively impacted her petitioning trips to Jinan and Beijing. Four years previously, one of Mali's neighbors was building a three-level building facing her yard. When she saw that she was to be overlooked by three big glass windows with a bird's-eye view of her flats and her yard, she was outraged. This meant that she and her family were entirely exposed to the neighboring family without any sense of privacy. She requested that the neighbor block the windows, but they refused. Finally she went to ask for justice at the residents' committee and when she met with no satisfaction there, she went to the street agency for mediation; no one wanted to intervene, however, as Mali's neighbor is a powerful manager of the local gas company.

Mali hovered around different government sectors in Zhangqiu, Shandong Province, including street agencies and the public security bureau, voicing her grievances and seeking help and justice. However, she was kicked around by these institutions, none of which wanted to get involved. Officials might read her documents, but at best they directed her to other government departments. Finally, she went to Jinan, the provincial capital, where her neighbor seemed to have connections as well. She was ignored by a series of *xinfang* offices. Once she was sitting in line at a *xinfang* office for three days for another chance to explain her case when she was forcibly returned by the police to the public security bureau in Zhangqiu, which further informed her street agency to take her back. In this process, she was labeled "psychotic." She was not, but she did suffer anxiety and depression because of the constant trips to different cities and manipulation at the hands of authorities, which took a toll on her physical and psychological well-being. However, with the prospect of exposing her family and private life to that bullying neighbor, she did not want to stop. Finally, she started to write petitioning letters to state leaders. After receiving no reply, she went to Beijing on a number of occasions, where she was perceived as crazy, as other petitioners often are, and she was several times put into the *shourong* (the Collecting Office for petitioners and homeless people). In telling me about her several years of petitioning experiences, she said,

It has been very exhausting, humiliating, and excruciating. You are treated as a paranoiac who is crazy to find fault with the government. ... Even healthy people can be tortured to be ill, physically and mentally. The folk saying "all petitioners are mentally ill" is not entirely untrue, but you are entirely tortured until you become crazy. The feeling of being wronged, bullied, manipulated, the feeling of vulnerability can really force you to act like a mad dog, as crazy as possible, to plead for justice, to retaliate. ... You cannot afford to stop, because you have sacrificed so much of your health, your finance, your time, but you cannot really win.

Eventually Mali received a letter from Qiao Shi, then director of the Central Political Bureau of the CCP. Much to her surprise, with this letter the local public security bureau finally intervened. The neighbor did block the windows facing her yard. But it took over four years of her valuable time. Her hair had entirely turned gray. While she was considered by *xinfang* officials at different levels as someone who may resemble the "litigious paranoiac" who has considerable legal knowledge, is a fanatical believer in her rights, and vehemently pursues her cause (Goldstein 1987), she indeed developed symptoms of depression and anxiety and suffered from serious insomnia.

Officials in charge of receiving and serving petitioners are not local governors. They have no power or resources to meet petitioners' pragmatic demands. What they often do is merely explain relevant policies and comfort the angry or frustrated petitioners. Still, many petitioners cannot accept "symbolic satisfaction." They continue to feel angry. Sometimes they lose patience and even beat up *xinfang* officials. To maintain a semblance of social order, officials have, therefore, developed a series of complex strategies to control petitioners, including manipulative actions that spark emotional responses.

One tactic is to confuse and defuse. As scholars have pointed out, some petitioners have a deep understanding of policies and can use them skillfully (O'Brien and Li 2006). Faced with such petitioners, officials adopt evasive tactics in an attempt to shift focus or confuse them. They *huo xini* – literally translated as "make soft dough" – dragging petitioners through endless procedures and exhausting them. But before a government leader offers a possible solution to a persistent petitioner, *xinfang* officials try to defuse petitioners' emotions to avoid conflicts and buy time for their leaders. In sum, the core function of *xinfang* work is not to solve conflicts, but to absorb potential protests

in non-violent ways that manipulate, obfuscate, and exhaust petitioners. The central issue is that while more and more people are desperate
for help (owing to dislocation and decreased local resources), the
bureaucracy is less and less responsive and the party state is ultimately
not held accountable.

### "UNEMPLOYMENT COMPLEX SYNDROME"

The sensational murder case on the eve of the opening ceremony of
the 2008 Beijing Olympic Games – a man who was reportedly unemployed and suffered from mental illness killed an American citizen –
showcased the default Chinese media representation that rationalizes
the association of unemployment with mental illness. The assumption
is that workers' job loss is due to mental illness rather than the other
way around (see J. Yang 2007, 2015). While such representations aim
to downplay the political motivation of retaliation crimes, they fore-
ground the psychological and emotional distress of those laid-off
workers. Indeed, Chinese psychologists have characterized the latest
wave of layoffs in medical terms, resulting in *shiye zonghezheng* (unemployment complex syndrome) (Wang 2008: 166), which is associated
with physical symptoms including hair loss, graying hair, and stomach-
ache, and psychological symptoms such as anxiety, depression, eating
disorders, and, potentially, suicide.

This unemployment syndrome is both a material condition and a
state- and expert-sponsored discourse legitimizing psychotherapy as
a solution to unemployment. "Unemployment complex syndrome"
pathologizes the reactions of workers coping with traumatic layoffs as
a result of state enterprise restructuring. Given the grim job market in
China, the constant pressure to look for re-employment exacerbates
these symptoms. Many workers I have spoken to in Changping have
conveyed, with extraordinary acuity, stories of trauma from layoffs and
its impact on their emotions and bodies. Some laid-off workers claimed

to have bombed their factories, while others have vandalized or stolen factory property in retaliation against these anti-working-class policies. In February 2002, a watch factory's warehouse was broken into and raw materials worth 200,000 RMB were stolen, despite there being four gate guards on duty that night. The police were certain that this involved unemployed workers as well as insider assistance (from some of the guards). In another instance, which has a humorous dimension to it, an agitated laid-off worker sought revenge by reporting the "death" of the factory party secretary to the local crematorium and asked for a corpse-collection van to be sent to this man's home. Suicide has also become more common as layoffs have increased. Since 1997, when layoffs were initiated in Changping because of the downsizing of the workforce, eight people at the watch factory where I have conducted fieldwork since 2002 have committed suicide. Most were men. Several left suicide notes indicating that layoffs were to blame.[2] It is socioeconomic conditions that have led to these deaths and to the increased attention to the psychology of the Chinese working class, and the pathologizing discourse of unemployment complex syndrome.

Since the mid-1990s, the downscaling and privatization of state-owned enterprises in China has resulted in the layoff of over 35 million workers and transformed more than 16 million of them into new urban poor (Rocca 2003). Workers' drastic downward mobility from Mao's elite to an urban underclass in recent years has precipitated social unrest. Indeed, for workers, being laid-off represents not only a loss of basic resources for subsistence but also a loss of status and identity. In Mao's era, unemployment was viewed as a typical product of capitalist societies, one that communism, which offers ways of overcoming capitalism, sought to eradicate. Within the all-encompassing work-unit system, people enjoyed guaranteed employment for life; unemployment did not exist, let alone unemployment complex syndrome.

Indeed, China's work units regulated both labor and residence. Labor relations at socialist work units were characterized by worker dependence and managerial paternalism (Walder 1986). Workers sup-posedly enjoyed cradle-to-grave welfare, known as the "iron rice bowl" (jobs for life in China's state sector). The working class used to be the vanguard, and that iron rice bowl – representing stable, long-term employment with a full state welfare package – made them the elite of the nation. This system is now fading. The loss of the iron rice bowl is evident in the degradation of status and living conditions among workers in China. Now flexibility is the buzzword. To be young, edu-cated, flexible, and "marketable" are the valued identity traits while stability is devalued.

Loss of status is at the heart of unemployment complex syndrome and of nostalgia for the iron rice bowl. Recently, however, rather than being viewed as a source of emotional, communal, and psychological support for urban workers, the iron rice bowl has been re-evaluated and criticized for inhibiting individual agency and productivity by increasing dependency on the state. Indeed, the fascination with the iron rice bowl, which is seen as contributing to unemployment complex syndrome, has been pathologized as an illness that needs to be treated. It is reported that a mother was cheated out of 2.06 million yuan by an employer in exchange for an "iron rice bowl" position for her son (Dong 2014). This amount of money is already more than enough to pay the salary for her young son until he retires. This example of someone who agreed to give up all her financial resources in order to secure the now uncommon guarantee of lifelong job security for her son may illuminate the tremendous significance of secure state jobs in people's outlooks and the traumatic effect on workers of layoffs from state enterprises (Solinger 2006; J. Yang 2007).

Because of unemployment complex syndrome and the understand-ing that growing unemployment posed a threat to the operation of the market economy and society, between 1995 and 2003, China under-took a national re-employment project. Since then, helping laid-off workers with re-employment has remained a priority for local governments and institutions. However, rather than focusing on job supply, the new re-employment framework has adopted an individualized and psychologized approach. Techniques of counseling and positive psychology have been integrated into these re-employment programs, with the aim of transforming the attitudes, emotions, and thought processes of the unemployed to help them adapt to the market economy (J. Yang 2015). What appears to be at issue is not attention to genuine psychological disorders, but, rather, permutations of psychological knowledge, modes of judgment, and forms of intervention for implementation with the unemployed. Class-based socioeconomic issues are transformed through these permutations into matters of individual emotions and psychology. For laid-off workers, unemployment complex syndrome does exist, but not because workers are maladaptive in the market economy or psychologically weak. Rather, these are people who have experienced job loss, disillusionment, and desperation owing to mass layoffs, which were carried out in ways that made them feel they were targeted by state enterprise restructuring, stripped of their identities and ways of making a living, and devalued in the new economy.

## "INTERNET ADDICTION"

China now is the biggest online gaming market in the world, surpassing the United States and Japan, with US$22 billion in revenue in 2015. China has the greatest number of Internet users in the world – 632 million as of July 2014 – and the government believes that 10 percent of its Internet-surfing minors (24 million) are addicted.[3] *Wangyin* (Internet addiction) is often associated with young students (18–30 years old, predominantly male) who are obsessed with surfing online or playing online games to an extent that prevents them from engaging with school or work. It is often treated at Internet addiction boot camps, where various forms of controversial "treatment," including brainwashing and electroconvulsive therapy, are implemented. However, the validity of this diagnosis, which China was the first country to uphold in 2008, is contested. Educators and psychiatrists argue that children's excessive use of the Internet is attributable to poor parenting rather than to a psychomedical disorder. Indeed, in the Fifth Edition of the *Diagnostic and Statistical Manual of Mental Disorders* (DSM-5), Internet addiction has been listed not as a disease category, but as a condition warranting more clinical research and experience before it might be considered for inclusion as a formal disorder.

In order to treat so-called Internet addiction, psychiatrist Yang Yongxin from Linyi, Shandong Province, administered a low-dose "electrical stimulus." Rather than curing the condition, however, this treatment, which inflicts great pain, may cause additional physical and psychological problems. While this therapy was banned in 2009 by China's Ministry of Health, it continues to be used to treat thousands of students each year. Yang, a self-claimed "national expert on Internet addiction," indicated that his innovative "wakeup brain therapy" involved 1~5 mA of current through the brain. While he acknowledged that this did cause pain, he claimed it was very safe. In his center for "quitting the Internet," patients had to take medications – including *yishu* and *leyou*, drugs for anxiety and depression three times a day.[4] Yang's use of electroconvulsive therapy to "punish" the person with Internet addiction is known as "aversion therapy," in which a punitive treatment is designed to eliminate maladaptive behavior. When the patient acts in undesired ways, he or she will be immediately given a certain degree of electroconvulsive therapy, producing a painful aversion response.

Similarly, another famous Internet addiction specialist, psychiatrist Tao Ran, a colonel in the People's Liberation Army, directs a militaristic rehab, the Daxing Internet Addiction Treatment Centre in Beijing (with about 250 spin-off camps throughout China), where "Internet addicts" are cut off from the outside world for three to six months with no web access or electronics and are forced to wear camouflage military attire and follow orders like soldiers. Anthropologist Trent Bax (2014) considers Tao Ran's methods a form of torture, contesting Tao's assertion that Internet addiction is comparable to drug addiction. Bax argues that withdrawal symptoms for Internet users are distinctive and are not linked to the taking of substances. He believes Internet addiction should be considered a social deviation rather than a medically "curable" condition.

In China, while psychiatrists like Yang Yongxin and Tao Ran treat obsessive use of the Internet as an addiction and a psychiatric disease comparable to alcohol or drug addiction, there are psychologists and educators who treat the addiction to the Internet as a social problem, reflecting issues in parenting, child–parent relationships, and the educational system. These experts argue that Internet addiction cannot be treated the same way as other psychiatric diseases, and liken the use of electroconvulsive therapy to cutting off one's hand to cure one's habitual masturbation (Tang 2016). Indeed, rather than curing the condition, this treatment, which inflicts great pain, may cause additional physical and psychological problems. It is reported to create a loss of interest in life that often presages serious depression and even suicide.

Through analysis of the lifeworld of those labeled "Internet addicts" in China, instead of pathologizing Internet addiction as a biomedically based behavior, Bax (2014) problematizes the relationship between Internet addicts and their social environment as dysfunctional. He contends that the Internet is not causing the addiction but represents a sanctuary where troubled youth seek solace and emotional escape. These "Internet addicts" are not pathological but living in a psycho-social-structural dilemma. Bax argues that while these "Internet-addicted" youth are viewed as having difficulty in both controlling their Internet use and normal social functioning, underneath this existential, ethical, and social crisis is a socially-economically-politically motivated competition: between China's educational system, expressed through schools and parents, and the larger consumer society, expressed through the online gaming industry oriented to transforming and individualizing the hearts and minds of China's youth.

There is also an alternative folk healing approach to Internet addiction in China. In my interviews with parents who went to MKH in Beijing and ZYH in Shandong Province, they claimed that the clinical treatment did little to relieve their children's addiction to the Internet but their determination and efforts to cure their children's addiction sometimes had positive effects in reducing their Internet access. One seemingly efficacious treatment I have learned of from two informants occurred through faith in Christianity and prayers. One of these informants went to consult a psychiatrist at ZYH about the Internet addiction of her son, a university student, but found the recommended treatment unsystematic and experimental (ZYH-2013-p12); a combination of medication and aversion therapy. Without alternative options and at her wits' end, she turned to Christian prayer when her son became so consumed by gaming that he would not answer the phone when she called him. The woman believes that her extensive prayer led to a positive change in her own attitudes toward her son and her son's behavior. She was later invited to offer a public testimony at her church to inspire other parents to turn to God to resolve their children's Internet addiction. She then organized a prayer group at the church to pray for other "Internet addicts."

These two approaches – aversion therapy and prayer therapy – emerge from the same willful ignorance of the stresses behind game addiction. These derive from the pressures of the utilitarian exam-centered educational system, which reduces the dynamics of young people's lives to a tedious grade-oriented existence (for further discussion on this subject, see below on *kongxin bing*). In turn, this situation is exploited by the booming and profitable gaming industry, which lures youth to consume and gain a sense of freedom. The various methods of treatment of Internet addiction only highlight the lack of treatment for structural ills, which, left unaddressed, give rise to increased distress.[5]

## "EMPTY-HEART DISEASE"

Xu Kaiwen (2016), deputy director of the Psychological Health Education and Counseling Center at Beijing University, uses *kongxin bing* (empty-heart disease) to describe a psychological disorder widespread among university students. *Kongxin bing* is attributed to the collapse of one's value orientation owing to external forces (in this context, China's educational system). It is not a strict diagnostic category, but its symptoms resemble those of depression, such as low spirits, indifference, unhappiness, and feelings of exhaustion, frustration, and meaninglessness that students experience as a consequence of their grade-driven life. Among first-year students at Beijing University, China's highest-ranked university, 40.4 percent reported feeling that life was meaningless, and 30.4 percent hated studying (Xu 2016).[6] However, according to Xu, these symptoms do not appear as severe as those of depression and are not sensitive to biomedical treatment, including the use of antidepressants, cognitive reconstruction, and electroconvulsive therapy. Indeed, biomedical factors are not closely associated with the symptoms of *kongxin bing*. Traditional psychotherapies are not efficacious either. Xu contends that it is China's utilitarian exam-centered educational system that induces feelings of mental distress among its students.

Bright signs with slogans that mobilize students to work hard for their university entrance exams hang at iron-barred high-school campuses, and anti-suicide scrutiny and surveillance create an impression of these campuses as both prisons and mental hospitals. Xu suggests that this kind of education can only produce students who require increasing sessions of counseling and never-ending crisis interventions after they enter universities. According to Xu, in 2015, Beijing

University's counseling center offered over 6,000 counseling sessions, while untold numbers of students are still waiting for their turns. The grade-oriented education trains students into "slaves" who do not know why they live except for high marks that temporarily give them a sense of achievement and success. Students' value orientations become twisted and opportunistic. Obtaining high marks and being admitted to famous universities have become the only driving force for their lives and the only criterion for their self-evaluation. Once these students have achieved their goals, they feel empty and do not know what life is for.

Those who suffer *kongxin bing* may not appear so different from "normal" students, but their inner experience is one of loneliness and meaninglessness. They lack significant connections with the world. They spend a tremendous amount of time on getting good grades, which, like drugs, cannot fill the emptiness and meaninglessness they experience. They may have good interpersonal relationships by striving to become good children and good students, but what they do is for other people, not for themselves, and thus they feel exhausted and futile rather than fulfilled. Many have strong suicidal tendencies, which derive not from difficulties or suffering in life but from a lack of purpose and meaning. These students live like walking corpses.

Parents are complicit in such opportunistic education, investing money and time to force their children to work hard at both school and after-school programs. Parents' own sense of worth seems tied to the success of their children, constructing the "networked" selves of the students in a negative way. In fact, after-school training, which parents often force their children to attend, not only further exhausts students but also exacerbates their relationship with their parents. Moreover, the grade-driven exam-based system collapses students' social support system as they see their peers as their rivals, constantly competing with them for a university place. Their lack of social support from their peers and worsened relationship with their parents together with the loss of their value orientation make these high school students vulnerable. Their subjectivity is based on grade-oriented and exam-centered education rather than on rich and concrete interpersonal relationships with peers and parents.

## CONCLUSION

This chapter has analyzed new mental illnesses created by psychologists and psychotherapists and reiterated by the public. I contend that these "illnesses" are not really individual psychological disorders but idioms of distress that express shifting social and cultural meanings in the context of socioeconomic dislocation in China. The pathologization of social issues or behaviors also partly results from the transformation of value and ethics since Mao's time. Take the so-called "workaholic" as an example. In Mao's era, there was no such a thing as workaholic as everyone was encouraged to dedicate themselves to work or politics rather than their personal lives. Only in the reform-era market economy has a balance of work and leisure been advocated for encouraging people to advance consumer capitalism; the putative balance of work and leisure, which would be considered bourgeois against the backdrop of the socialist collective ethics in Mao's era, is now treasured as a type of cosmopolitan lifestyle guided by an emphasis on individual-centered ethics. Moreover, the pathologization of social phenomena as individual illness promotes therapeutic strategies, nurturing happiness and self-fulfillment to further enhance (therapeutic) consumption and develop the mental health industry.

In general, psychologists, psychiatrists, and the public are encouraged to recognize new forms of craziness or novel illnesses in service of the booming psychotherapy industry. The pathologization and psychologization of social issues is promoted by the psychoboom in Chinese society. Foucault (1976) suggests psychology has constructed madness. Indeed, the categories of Internet addiction, empty-heart disease, petitioning bigotry, princess disease, country bumpkin syndrome and unemployment complex syndrome are examples of the extension of the frontiers of psychology into previously non-commercial, non-medical territories of ordinary social intercourse.

With the individualization and psychologization of social problems in China, structural forces that contribute to social problems are manifested in personal emotions, individual struggles, and psychological discourses. Consequently, blame is sought in the individual, rather than in the systematic transformations that create severe contradictions, injustice, and frustrating barriers within people's lives.

# Gender, Class, and Mental Health

_____

The stronger and the more controlling the mother is, the more she will be
detrimental to the family.

*Wu Xi'an 2016*

To interpret as illness [women's] routinized forms of suffering and
experiences of deprivation is to medicalize and thereby trivialize and
distort the significance of societal oppression.

*Kleinman and Kleinman 1994*

Women are overrepresented in Chinese official statistics on mental
disorders such as suicide, schizophrenia, and eating disorders (Pearson
1995; Lee and Lee 2000; Phillips 2001; Jackson and Chen 2007).[1]
Multiple explanations have been put forward for this gender gap. It may
be due to women's marginal status, gendered differences in attitudes
toward admitting vulnerability and seeking help, or differences in the
delivery of mental health services to men and women (Pearson 1995;
Busfield 2012). Because gender configures men's and women's material
and symbolic positions in the social hierarchy, as well as their experiences of and responses to such inequalities, it sets up preconditions for
good health. In the case of mental health globally, gender is considered
a health determinant that interacts with other key factors, including
class, to define access to resources and treatment (WHO 2002). As the
second quote at the start of this chapter highlights, differences in mental
health between men and women index and reinforce their unequal positions in society. To understand women's needs for and use of mental

health services requires a fuller account of the negative social situations that women experience. In this chapter, I conduct a feminist analysis of ethnographic data from China to explore socioeconomic inequalities as a major factor contributing to the higher incidence of women's mental distress, and the way social hierarchies and inequalities affect the lives of women and men and their experiences of mental distress.

The relationship between gender and mental distress is "not fixed or universal; rather, as gender relations change, including gendered differences in status, power, resources, opportunities, and cultural expectations," so does the mental health profile of a community or nation (Busfield 2012: 205). Gender itself is heavily influenced by social, economic, and cultural processes, and there are clear cross-cultural differences in the way it is conceptualized (Patel 2005). Mental distress is also shaped by cultural and regional factors (Kleinman 1987). Phyllis Chesler (1972: 56) contends that gender is encompassed in the very definition of mental distress: what is considered "madness," whether it appears in women or in men, is "either the acting out of the devalued female role or the total or partial rejection of one's sex role stereotype." Chesler suggests that a gender asymmetry exists in which women are more likely to be identified as disturbed than men; while many men are also severely "disturbed," the forms their disturbances take are either not seen as neuroses or are not treated by residential psychiatric care. In China, gender is central in its transformation from a socialist planned economy to a market economy. Women suffer from the effects of the country's economic restructuring to a greater extent than men, for instance through unemployment and diminished public support in education and child care.

An example from my ethnographic research in Changping illustrates this point. After her layoff from a factory there in 2007, a woman worker named Ren committed suicide by walking into traffic on a highway. At her funeral, the director of the watch factory where she had been employed indicated that she had always looked *shenshen daodao* (superstitious and secretive), implying she was not adequately social or "normal." However, almost all the woman's co-workers I interviewed pointed to her layoff rather than an introverted personality as the catalyst for her suicide.

Ren had once been publicly scolded by her workshop director for an error in processing watch parts and was first to be laid off at her workshop as privatization began, a loss of both "face" and identity for her within her community (see Chapter 2 on "unemployment complex syndrome"). During the two weeks back home after her layoff, Ren grew more silent and more subdued. Her husband did not pay much attention to her low spirits as he did not know what exactly had happened at work. In this case, job loss and lack of social support likely contributed to Ren's suicide, although officials referenced a "flawed" personality, attaching blame to individual character rather than socioeconomic change. In Changping, in fact, more men than women have taken their own lives following massive layoffs. Yet Ren's suicide was the only one attributed by factory management to introversion and *xiang bu kai* (inability to think out). In general in Changping, women's mental distress and suicide are more likely to be attributed to personality or psychological states than to frustration about socioeconomic difficulties, which are more often associated with men's suicide and mental distress. This distinction in perceived causes of mental distress influences mental health care and poverty-relief programs, which tilt toward benefiting men more than women. This imbalance, in turn, relates to a deeper issue of how working-class masculinity is perceived by the state; disgruntled laid-off men are perceived to represent a threat to social stability and, therefore, they are treated in a more accommodating fashion than are their female counterparts (see J. Yang 2010, 2015).

Indeed, social responses to mental distress show gendered differences in perception, with greater stigma and rejection attaching to women who suffer mental illness. However, identifying gender differences in the incidence of mental disorders is not enough. Gender differences affect the definitions of men's and women's mental distress, their respective risks and vulnerabilities, their access to health services, and the social and economic consequences of mental illness in different settings and social groups and at different points in the life cycle (cf. Patel 2005). This chapter explores observed gender differences in the definition, distribution, and treatment of mental disorders in China and how the state utilizes these gendered differences for its own social, economic, and political purposes. I argue that the emergence of essentialized psychological discourses, by psychologizing gendered differences and deviations from gender norms, conceals the structural roots of distress. These discourses reinforce psychological stereotypes against women (including fixing women in the domestic sphere and their roles of wife and mother) and create new forms of social exclusion.

## GENDERED PSYCHOLOGY AND ESSENTIALIZED GENDER ROLES

Since the end of the 1970s, there has been a shift in gender ideology in China. During Mao's era, the government sought to downplay biological differences between men and women to masculinize women and maximize the use of their labor. Today, the situation is reversed: the state emphasizes biological differences, promoting a naturalized or even essentialized view of gender and highlighting hyperfemininity (and domestic femininity). One of the most obvious effects of this shift has been women's retreat from the public sector to the domestic sphere, which has widened the income gap between husbands and wives, lowering women's status and diminishing their control over their own lives, marriages, and reproductive events. Meanwhile, China's beauty industry has exploited the focus on feminine beauty, feminine youth, and sexual submissiveness (Yang 2011b). Thinness, as a quality in women appealing to men, is now highly valued, leading to an increase in eating disorders among young Chinese women (see Jackson and Chen 2008).

Among those who are aged between 30 and 39, professional women, who experience more pressure at work and from interpersonal relationships, as well as from the raising of children, especially children's education, reportedly have a higher incidence of depression than men, while women who hold middle-ranking managerial jobs suffer from greater work pressure than do ordinary employees.[2]

China's vast psychological self-help literature, which people might turn to as a remedy for distress, is also gendered. This literature and associated media, including books, websites, and counseling services, tend to essentialize gender and attribute certain psychological traits to each of the sexes. For instance, Chinese counselors see a sense of security as vital to women's physical and mental health and yet acknowledge a lack of security as epidemic among women in the country (Li 2016). Accordingly, women suffer from stress, anxiety, and depression, which can affect other aspects of their health and their identities as well. By contrast, Chinese counselors consider a sense of "lacking recognition" to be epidemic among males. When men do not have an identity that gives them self-recognition, they search for recognition from others close to them; a "weak wife" can serve this purpose. Some men feel a lack of control if their wife is in an equal professional position to them. It is only through a wife's submission that such a man bolsters his own sense of self. This stereotype reinforces the gendered expectations that women cannot be as strong-willed and as capable and successful as men. Men's pursuit of "face" is described as a way of seeking social recognition; those who eagerly seek "face" usually lack a sense of self-recognition (Li 2016). However, Ren's experience of a lack of "face" when she was laid off offers a counter-example, which highlights how these essentializing discourses fail to capture the socioeconomic pressures affecting men and women today.

The well-known Chinese counselor Li Zixun (2016) promotes such essentializing views of men's and women's psychological traits and emotional lives. Men, he argues, are keen to use reason, power, and violence to control and even break apart the world, while women use their water-like emotions to repair the world. For Li, in a world dominated by men, a woman may suffer from depression owing to inner conflict: should she pursue her own goals or submit to masculine and rational power? If she embraces independence, she will pay a price; such a woman is often viewed as "disturbed" by society. If she submits to male power, she is trapped in a weak role. Li nevertheless concludes that women accommodate the maintenance of male interest and affection. If men represent the "natural" power of human beings via aggression, dominance, and expansion, then women represent humanity's inner nature through management, governance, and tolerance.

This discourse follows a typical media pattern opposing women to men in China, with men as the foil and standard and women developing psychologically to serve men's interests, as well as, by extension, those of the family and state. The implied pedagogy for women is "how to become a woman whom a man cannot live without," "a woman who makes her husband flourish." In this pedagogy, women also learn how to become "wise mothers" and "virtuous wives" and to make a whole family happy, healthy, and successful, implicitly contributing to a harmonious society. Conversely, *qiangshi muqin* (strong-willed mothers) are pathologized alongside *yiyu de muqin* (depressed mothers). In an article titled "The Stronger and the More Controlling the Mother is, the More She Will be Detrimental to the Family," Wu Xi'an (a male author) (2016) argues that women who are strong-willed and garrulous do harm to their children's personality development and to familial harmony: "The more strong-willed and more controlling the mother is, the weaker her son becomes and the more overbearing her daughter will be." Characteristics of such controlling mothers include self-righteousness, self-centeredness, fault-finding, and dictating. These women are said to lack a sense of security, base their self-value on the approval of others, and lack trust in their husbands. Wu proposes that a wise mother gives her husband more opportunities to educate their children and more say in their children's lives, while respecting her husband in front of the children. The psychological discourse reinforces the value of sacrifice, docility, and submissiveness for women, just as China relaxes its one-child family policy and many women are deciding on a second child, requiring happy and well-adjusted mothers.

Epidemiological data from the 1960s and 1970s typically show that mental illness has been more common in women than men, which supports the feminist claim that the gender division of labor disadvantaged women (Busfield 2012). According to Richard Cloward and Frances Piven (1979), the way people respond to stress is socially constructed; these responses are channeled by the normative rules of society and are socially regulated. Hence, it is useful to attend to the cognitive and moral framework through which stresses are interpreted. Resources, cultural expectations, and essentializing discourses have encouraged women either to passively endure stress or to engage in individualistic self-destructive forms of deviance. In particular, Cloward and Piven contend that the rise of the health care system leads women to view the tensions they experience as rooted in their physical or mental health and to search within their psyches and their bodies for the source of their problems. Not only are women encouraged to think this way, but their employers and the public also tend to attribute their mental distress to the individuals and their personalities, as illustrated in Ren's suicide in Changping. In contrast, male deviance tends to be more collectively oriented and to involve violence and aggression against others (Pearson 1995; cf. Busfield 2012).

A contrast thus emerges between turning feelings inward (often attributed to women) and turning them outward. This idea breaks down the strategy for dealing with distress into internalization (subjection of the person to the standards of others) and externalization (turning feelings outward, especially aggression) (Busfield 2012). Indeed, psychiatrists now often talk of two types of psychological disorders: internalizing disorders, typified by anxiety and depression, which are more common in women, and externalizing disorders, typi-fied by aggressive and antisocial behavior, but also including substance abuse disorders, for example alcohol-triggered violence and aggression, which are more common in men (Pearson 1995; Busfield 2012). While such differences may be influenced by genetic factors, they also relate to the socialization of women and men in childhood – socialization that is linked to gendered expectations in adult life. Differences in women's and men's socioeconomic situations have a direct impact on the gendered expression of feelings in the face of life events and difficul-ties (Busfield 2012, 2014).

## CLASS, GENDER, AND MENTAL DISTRESS

Scholars have suggested that stressful life events and chronic strains have an adverse impact on health, and that the frequency of such events increases as one moves lower on the socioeconomic scale (Mirowsky and Ross 2003). A link between social class and mental illness has long been established (Hollingshead and Redlich 1958), and similar ideas permeate discussions of gender differences in mental health (Busfield 2012). Most studies show an association between indicators of poverty and the risk of mental disorders. Factors such as the experience of insecurity and hopelessness, and the risks of violence and physical illness, may explain the greater vulnerability of the poor to mental disorders. Direct and indirect costs of mental illness also worsen peo-ple's economic standing, setting up a vicious cycle of poverty and mental disorder (Patel and Kleinman 2003; Zhang Jin 2016). In one study of four low- to middle-income countries undergoing rapid economic change, rising income disparities and economic inequality, being gen-dered as female, having low education, and living in poverty were strongly associated with common mental disorders, such as anxiety and depression (Patel et al. 1999). It is clear that structural effects of marginalization are often common to women and those lower on the socioeconomic ladder. To interpret as illness their routinized forms of suffering and experiences of deprivation is to medicalize and thereby trivialize and distort the significance of societal oppression (Kleinman and Kleinman 1991).

One day in July 2013 at Dr. Wen's office in ZYH, I met a woman in her mid-fifties named Gong (ZYH-2013-p3) and her husband. Gong's husband took her there because of her insomnia, nighttime crying, and sleepwalking. Dr. Wen asked whether any significant events had taken place in Gong's life recently, to which the husband replied that Gong's mother had passed away one month before. Gong snapped back that her husband had a secret mistress and was spending all his savings on her. Dr. Wen, who did not have time to hear the whole story, prescribed Gong medication for insomnia and anxiety. Hospitals in China often *yi yao yang yi* (subsidize medical services with paid drug prescriptions) and psychiatrists thus prescribe drugs much more often than they offer talk therapy.

Later, during a three-hour interview, Gong told me about her life and her distress. She once worked at a fabric factory, which had gone bankrupt ten years before. She had then found temporary work at the local park, making 800 RMB a month, which was not much but sufficient for her and her son's daily expenses. Her husband worked at a Zibo railway station, making about 4,500–5,500 yuan per month. He seldom gave her money for domestic use, but paid their son's college tuition. He also claimed to have been saving money for their son's wedding and first home, a normative practice in Zhangqiu. About three months before Gong's visit at ZYH, her son, now a public servant, announced that his girlfriend was pregnant and that they planned to marry soon. Gong immediately discussed this with her husband and expected him to help their son purchase an apartment. However, much to her surprise, her husband only produced RMB 70,000, allegedly his total savings. Gong was outraged, asking where he had spent his salary all these years, during which she had not asked him for a penny. She suspected that her husband must have spent his money on a mistress, as he only returned home once every two or three weeks. She was highly disillusioned with her own decision to bring up her son single-handedly, not relying on her husband for anything. She had changed the bulbs, carried heavy gas tanks, and performed other work usually undertaken by men in Zhangqiu.

Gong then went to her husband's workplace in Zibo and spoke with his boss about her husband's lifestyle. Her husband was ashamed by this loss of "face" before his employers and colleagues. Since then, Gong had been waking nightly, sometimes screaming, sometimes wailing, or waking her husband up for a fight. Unable to leave her to attend work, her husband had brought her back to ZYH to find a solution. While both her husband and Dr. Wen believed that she suffered from mental illness, Gong did not think she was ill, but rather deeply disappointed, angry, and deflated after years of hard work and juggling a disciplined and frugal life. Her mother's passing, and the prospect of becoming a mother-in-law and grandmother, had added to her stress. Gong deeply regretted not handling her husband's income sooner, but even more, she regretted that she had not enjoyed life as much as her husband had. While she never discovered a mistress, she did learn from her husband's colleagues that he had always had a comfortable lifestyle, dining out and dressing well. He never expressed guilt about not helping his wife with domestic responsibilities. It then came to Gong that she and her husband did not come from the same class: her husband led a middle-class lifestyle, while she had lived with the frugal mentality typical of the urban underclass, especially after her layoff. Social support may serve as a buffer between deleterious social circumstances and developing depression or neurotic disorders (Miles 1987), but in Gong's case, she lacked her husband's support while bringing up her son and coping with life amidst dwindling economic resources.

When asked to explain what is attributed to their mental distress, most of my informants offer social accounts (cf. Pearson 1995). While surface symptoms often include insomnia, poor appetite, dizziness, and headaches, further questioning elicits deeper emotional and social difficulties, which they and their families, but not necessarily doctors, link directly to the distress. At the same time, diagnosis of only the medical symptoms can be beneficial to Gong. Being "ill" exempted her from normal duties: Gong stopped performing domestic tasks and stopped living a frugal life. Blame was imputed to Gong's husband by her family. Gong also received attention for her years of sacrifice that otherwise had been ignored. This diagnosis also benefited her husband and the psychiatrist if Gong was less combative and slept better and if she was consuming drugs.

For Gong, her socialization as a woman in a small town and as a working mother and wife had cultivated her habitual sacrifice of her own interests for her child and husband. Her lack of education and lower income and social status than her husband, especially after she had been laid off from the state sector, contributed to her subordination to him and lack of control over family affairs, giving rise to her frustration and despair in times of significant life events like her son's marriage. In general, as a member of the working class, Gong's downward mobility as a result of China's economic restructuring diminished her livelihood and widened the income gap between her and her husband, while medicine treated the symptoms of her anger and regret. Social disadvantage exacerbates distress while medicine can treat only biomedical symptoms, rather than alleviating structural injustices that likely contribute to the distress.

## PATHOLOGIZING "UNHAPPY, DEPRESSED MOTHERS"

According to the 2012 China Family Panel Studies survey, which included 40,000 respondents from 25 Chinese provinces, the gender difference in the prevalence rates of depression is striking. Not only were there fewer females in the mentally healthy group in comparison with males (45.74 percent vs. 57.68 percent), but many more female respondents were in the severe depression group (29.29 percent vs. 18.66 percent) (Qin et al. 2015).

The age and gender hierarchy that typifies Chinese society frequently means that there is still limited autonomy for women regarding decisions, for example, about employment and abortion. Feeling a lack of autonomy and control over one's life is known to be associated with depression (Pearson 1995). Further, women are socialized to be "other-oriented" (Horwitz et al. 1996), resulting in a tendency to concern themselves with interpersonal relationships. The relational form of selfhood that exists in China also contributes to Chinese women's concern about others, especially family members. Therefore, women are more vulnerable to the stresses of deprivation of interpersonal ties and, as a result, to depression. Suppression of emotions has also been found to be relevant to Chinese women's experiences of suffering. Veronica Pearson and Meng Liu (2002) suggest that suicidal women are often vulnerable because they experience difficulty in constructively expressing their anger within rigid social and family structures. The Confucian values of obedience and submission among Chinese women in relation to men may also play a crucial role in this restriction of emotional expression (Hsiao et al. 2006).

The gender gap in depression, in which women suffer more, has been demonstrated in community-based studies around the world (Patel et al. 1999). Stress is a known factor that can lead to depression, and greater exposure to stressors may partly explain excessive risk for depression among women. In China, the rate of depression among those *tekun qunti* (groups in extreme difficulty) whose livelihood heavily relies on the social safety net is often seven times higher than those who do not rely on it (Zhang Jin 2016). More women relative to men are affected by poverty and downward social mobility in the lower classes in China than in the middle class. Further, growing evidence now associates economic difficulties with a higher risk for depression (Patel and Kleinman 2003); the social gradient in health is heavily gendered, and women are disproportionately affected by the burden of poverty, which, in turn, may influence their vulnerability for depression. Women are also far more likely to be victims of violence in their homes; those who experienced physical violence by an intimate partner are significantly more likely to suffer depression, abuse drugs, or attempt suicide (Patel et al. 1999).

The association between gender, class, and mental disorders is evident in Changping, a working-class community that experienced mass unemployment owing to economic restructuring starting in the mid-1990s. This triggered a rise in alcoholism among laid-off male workers, as well as domestic violence against women, and depression and suicide among women. One of my informants, named Lan, came to Changping with her mother 20 years ago from Henan Province. Her mother later remarried to a male worker from the local watch factory. Much to everyone's surprise, the next year, Lan married her stepbrother, who is 10 years older than her. Later, it turned out that she married him because he had raped her; her mother was worried about her reputation and marriage was a ready solution. The rape and marriage had tremendous mental health consequences for Lan, however. She was depressed, though she did not get a formal diagnosis until she attempted suicide after she gave birth to her son. In retrospect, the psychosocial workers in her community believed that her original depression probably worsened owing to a postpartum disorder. Her husband was not supportive during this period of worsening depression. After his layoff in 2003, he drank more, squandering his meager earnings as a taxi-driver, rather than regularly taking his wife to MKH to see her psychiatrist. The director of the local residents' committee constantly scolded him to live up to what he had promised to his wife, and reminded him of his responsibility for his wife's mental distress. His mother-in-law was left to care for

Lan. She, in turn, complained to local authorities about her husband's neglect.

Lan's story provides insight into the social, class, and gendered aspects of distress, and also shows how gendered differences exist in care for mental patients. While a woman is required to become the primary caregiver if her husband is mentally ill, her own family is responsible for her care if she is stricken. Lan's case also exemplifies the mental health consequences of sexual violence, and the potential contribution of reproductive events to mental disorders. Indeed, genetic and biological factors (i.e., mood swings related to hormonal changes as a part of the menstrual cycle) may play some role in the higher prevalence of depressive and anxiety disorders among women (Pearson 1995). In the case of antenatal and postnatal depression, the interaction of psychosocial factors with hormonal factors appears to result in an elevated risk. Thus, as in Lan's case, marital disharmony, inadequate social support, and a poor financial situation are associated with an increased risk of postnatal depression.

Yet many prominent psychologists in China today attribute almost all psychological disorders to early childhood experience, especially the relationship to an unqualified, depressed mother (Li 2016; Wu Zhihong 2016). In this discourse, the mother is depicted as working outside the home, using daycare, and spending little time with her children. The resulting separation becomes a source of psychological distress for the child, including a sense of insecurity and a feeling of lack of love. In this vein, inner child therapy, which guides adults back through time to locate the ultimate sources of distress, pathologizes mothers who either work or otherwise separate from the infant.

This discourse legitimizes the gendered aspect of mass layoffs in China since the mid-1990s, which saw more rapid job losses for women than for men. The rationale is simply that "women should go home" (Wang 2003; Yang 2007). In short, the key message underlining the discourse of *yiyu de muqin* (depressed mothers) is that home can hurt, and the one who hurts is ultimately the mother. Even when fathers hurt their children, mothers are still to blame for being indifferent, or for their inability to intervene.

This discourse is powerful enough to impact people's perceptions of their relationships with working mothers. The following example from my ethnography illustrates how one woman participated in dance therapy (an offshoot of inner child therapy) in order to deal with negative feelings about her mother, whom she perceived as absent. I spoke to her after a dance therapy session in Beijing in the summer of 2015 in which she had participated. She is an aspiring counselor and the mother of two teenage boys. She did the dance therapy session alone and described to me how she benefited from it.

> I started to dance freely. No audience, no performance. It was my body speaking with the flow of the music. … Bending myself, my hands were reaching the ground waving. I waved to the earth, trying to get something from it or trying to give something to the earth. Then I slowly stood up with two hands giving something to the earth. All of a sudden I felt sad, hearing something from my heart, "Mom, I cannot give you anything." Then my eyes became misty. During the last three decades, I seemed always to try to save my mother. I wished her happiness and wealth. However, I cannot give her anything … .
>
> The music was flowing, … I lay down sticking to the ground. In my vision, I saw countless stems and roots growing up from the earth and they grasped me securely. … I heard another shout from my heart: Mom, I need you! Mom, I need you! Mom, I need you. I was shouting in my heart with tears streaming down quietly. I saw a small infant. … She was crying looking for her mother. Gradually, she realized that it was useless to cry. Mom was not there. Then she knew to take back her needs and started to smile at others. I picked up this infant gently, and told her, "Sweetie, you are so perfect; you're a gift from Heaven." … Mom put you here because she loves you. She wants to give you the

best of life. She needs to work to raise you. This is love, not abandonment. ... This dance therapy session surprised me: I truly heard my
body speaking. The body seems to be more intelligent and sensitive
than the mind, [I am] trusting it.

This account offers a two-part narrative: the first part is the woman's
realization of her vulnerability to her mother's issues, her mother's
unhappiness and lack of fulfillment. She worked hard but did not feel
fulfilled since, in Mao's era, women commonly coped with a double
shift both at work and at home (see Yang 1999). This becomes manifest in the second part of the story: owing to her mother's work,
the baby was left at daycare, alienated and wounded. Through her
body movements, the woman engaged in a dialogue with this unhappy
inner infant, comforting and healing it. The dance therapy session
both exposed this woman's deep wound and partially healed her. Her
narrative implicitly condemns the negative effects of women who
work outside the home on the psychological health of both themselves and their children. In this sense, psychology offers a "scientific
reason" legitimizing the recent emphasis on domestic femininity and
hyperfemininity, especially in the wake of massive "gendered layoffs"
(Wang 2003). This pathologizing discourse is apparently significant
for the Chinese government today, since happy, well-adjusted mothers
are particularly needed as China is on its way to relaxing its one-child
family planning policy. Women are ready to produce a second child for
the family and the state to revitalize an aging population in China. In
general, this discourse reinforces women's positions at home and in the
private sector. It confines a woman's happiness and liberation entirely
to the context of family and her relationship with her children and
husband.[3]

Weighing in on unhappy and depressed mothers, popular psychological self-help media in China construct an image of "happy housewives" and "happy mothers" (see Yang forthcoming). For instance, in

one article, Chinese success studies guru Chen Anzhi (2016) argues that a mother's personality determines whether her children are outstanding or not. Thus, mothers must strive to be happy and leave negative emotions outside before returning home. The worst scenario is if a mother transfers her bad heart-emotions to her children. Of course, this threat of ruining the family through unhappiness promotes therapeutic consumption; women are encouraged to gain a sense of happiness and fulfillment through purchasing things for the home and family. Indeed, happiness has emerged as a culturally and historically specific psychotherapeutic tool for governance of gender (particularly of marginalized women) in China (Yang 2014).

Self-help media mobilize women to play a vanguard role in promoting and performing "happiness." Through a woman's happiness the needs of men can be met. This is less an economic conspiracy directed against women and more something that happens to women when the business of producing, selling, and investing is organized to serve men's needs efficiently (cf. Friedan 1965). Happiness becomes a mode of subject formation. It derives from human agency, and the power to seek happiness is a mode of self-governance that can be co-opted for broader political and economic ends. By tapping into women's desires for happiness and enjoyment in everyday life, and addressing the potential locked in their domestic femininity, counseling programs and self-help genres mobilize women for entrepreneurship and consumerism. While "naturalizing" psychology as a method to free the self, such psychological self-help media also instill in women a specific sort of expert interpretation of who they are and what they want as wives and mothers. The rhetoric and imagery compel people (women in particular), whether explicitly or subliminally, to associate their behaviors and thoughts with self-imposed states of happiness and well-being, thereby achieving an element of social control. In this way, psychology oppresses women by rendering their emotions, hearts, and internal lives sites of regulation and value extraction.

## "THE SICK-MAN PHENOMENON": MASCULINITY AND DEPRESSION

It is impossible to consider the relationship between gender, class, and mental distress by only focusing on women's experience. Men suffer distress too, and their particular experience of distress interacts with social values as well as women's identity and feelings. I want to briefly survey a few popular perceptions of men's distress in China today. One is *nanren bing* (the sick-man phenomenon), which occurs predominantly among middle-class men. This phenomenon resembles depression, but has some uniquely Chinese characteristics related to masculinity. Counselor Xu Chunxia blames the sick-man phenomenon on mainstream social values such as the expectation that men should embody strength and be admired and served by women (Fan 2016). Linked to traditional culture, this form of masculinity rejects indications of softness or delicacy, as well as failure. Men learn to subdue their emotions, relying on forbearance and avoidance. When marital problems occur, women seek help, while most men endure them or escape by filing for divorce or indulging in extramarital affairs.

The incapacity of men to express emotion adeptly may lead to the incidence of *weixiao yiyu* (smiling depression) in China (Gao and Liu 2016). Men are shamed for expressing their emotions and tend to hide depression. This situation may also increase men's dependence on women for many aspects of domestic life. These factors contribute to high levels of distress among men when faced with loss, such as bereavement. According to the familiar sayings, men must not cry in public (*nan'er you lei bu qing tan*); men can shed blood but not tears (*nan'er liu xue bu liu lei*); and men fear nothing, neither heaven nor hell (*nan zi han tian bu pa di bu pa*). For many Chinese men, "silence is golden," making it difficult to know whether they are depressed. Men's silence, moreover, creates difficulties in husband–wife relationships, leaving them without good cues as to their spouses' states of mind. If men are raised in accordance with the norms crystalized in these folk sayings, it is hard for them to keep open communication with their parents. For some, including well-known counselor Wu Zhihong (2016), this results in adult men with immature personalities who are more or less "giant infants" who require therapy but do not know how to seek help. Data show that, as late as 2015, very few men sought help for emotional distress; among participants in online counseling or advice-seeking for emotional issues, less than 5 percent were men. A survey conducted in 2016 by Yi Xinli, an online psychological service platform, indicates that in China, women are the main clients for counseling; the ratio between female and male clients is 7:3.[4] Suicide has long been a way out for men in despair, a means to maintain the "tough guy" image. According to an international survey, the suicide rate of male patients with depression is much higher than it is for women. Among the 350 million patients with depression globally in 2011, the suicide rate for male patients was 78.5 percent (He 2016).

Because of instability as a result of its rapid formation, the Chinese middle class has been making efforts to distinguish itself from the lower classes through constructing a distinct identity (Goodman 2014). While those in the middle class appear to enjoy economic security, political detachment, and apparent privilege, they experience widespread anxiety and crises derived from their distrust of or sense of insecurity about the insufficient and inefficient social infrastructure in China: the lack of a social security system, for example (Jiang 2016). They suffer from tension, stress, and insomnia, often associated with *guo lao si* (overwork death). Many of them succumbed to *xiangpi ren* (literally "plasticine people" or "modeling-clay people," describing the condition of those who experience numbness, hopelessness, low spirits, and a loss of passion in life). It is considered as a type of depression that many Chinese middle-class men reportedly suffer, similar to the Western concept of job burnout. Chinese counselors often pathologize those who suffer from *xiangpi ren* as such conditions reduce the productivity and entrepreneurship expected of middle-class men (J. Yang 2015, 2016).

Mainly a condition of white-collar male workers, those who experience *xiangpi ren* are amenable and kneaded this way and that. Like plasticine, they are malleable, and like plastic casings, they are insulated, numb, and senseless. They are perceived to do things without thinking and to lose their ability for critical thinking. They have no dreams, ideals, or interests, and feel neither pain nor joy. Their motto is "one day at a time." Typically, they work alone for more than 50 hours a week. Women are underrepresented as suffering from *xiangpi ren*, owing to the assumption that it is "normal" and "natural" for women to be quiet, submissive, and flexible, or to lack energy. Members of the working class are also underreported in this category, in part because private counseling, which might lead to discovery of this phenomenon, remains a privilege of urban middle-class people.[5] This phenomenon of *xiangpi ren* partly explains the reason for women's distress, for it suggests that men pull out of social relationships and give up on others as their experiences of distress intensify. This creates a situation in which women lack the social support they need at home or at work (if they are working with men).

EATING DISORDERS

As *xiangpi ren* and "smiling depression" are phenomena attributed to men, which align them with the stereotypically caregiving and emotionally expressive qualities of women, disordered eating is perceived as a women's problem, but involves regimes of femininity that align with men's putative low interest in (facial) appearances. The "cult of thinness" has been increasingly propagated in China by books and magazines advocating weight-reducing diets, the fashion industry, which caters mainly to the slimmer figure, and television, which attaches sexual allure and professional success to the possession of a svelte physique (Russell 2000). The emphasis on women's thinness by the media and fashion industries is now leading to a rise in disordered eating in non-Western cultures, including China, as globalization leads to increasing homogenization of media imagery across the world, with Western imagery being the predominant force.

In Asian societies, a profound and dramatic shift in gender roles is underway based on economic pressures, a developing consumer culture, including globalized fashion and beauty industries, as well as media influence and acculturation (Pike and Dunne 2015). In China, eating disorders have been on the rise (Lee and Lee 2000; Jackson and Chen 2007, 2008; Björkell 2011; Pike and Dunne 2015). Zhang Darong, one of the first eating disorder specialists in China, who has been studying the issue since the early 1980s with Peking University's Sixth Hospital, indicates that the rate of anorexia nervosa has outpaced the country's capacity to understand or deal with the disorder. Most Chinese are unfamiliar with the term, and many hear about it for the first time when they are diagnosed. According to Zhang, there were only 52 eating disorder cases in the hospital from 1983 to 2001. By 2006, they dealt with that same number of patients each year. These days, they see about 20 patients every month (Liu 2012). There are therefore not enough treatment options for most people. While eating disorders are mostly viewed as a modern "female malady," there is an increasing incidence of these disorders among males because of changing cultural expectations for the "metrosexual" male.

Although much of the research on body image problems in non-Western countries suggests that increased exposure to Western media and Western ideals of attractiveness explains the rise of eating disorders in China (Jackson and Chen 2007), I focus on the way indigenous categories and conceptions of the female body may contribute to these disorders. For example, unlike in the West, where many women pay excessive attention to fitness, in China, dissatisfaction with one's face is a significant trigger for eating disorders (see Jackson and

Chen 2008). Thinness in the face (or a smaller, oval-shaped face) has been viewed as a key factor in determining a young woman's beauty and her marketability in the marriage market, or in determining whether one is photogenic or not. Many cellphone photo software applications in China can make people's faces look thinner, paler, and prettier.

The emphasis on facial appearance has a moral and gendered connotation in traditional folk knowledge regarding the role of facial structure and features in determining one's destiny. However, there has been a transformation in what is perceived as the ideal face and appearance to make a husband flourish (*wang fu*). Previously a woman desired a strong and plump face, but today a thin, oval face is thought to attract a rich husband. Whereas images of robust, working-class women signaled achievement in Mao's era, today the same message is conveyed by narrow chins and concave waists. Recently, scores of women posted photos on Chinese social media to prove their waists did not protrude from behind a vertical 8.3 × 11.7 inch piece of paper. The *People's Daily*, the Communist Party's flagship newspaper, called it a "fitness challenge." This phenomenon is also informed by its historical background: the only children who are the legacy of China's one-child policy tend to feel intense pressure to achieve success, good marriages, and better economic standing, which disposes them to turn to their culture for clues for achieving this success (Björkell 2011). The beauty economy is there to capitalize on the intensity of their desire. It focuses on feminine youth, feminine facial beauty, and female sexuality, and contributes to the construction of ideal female body images that today have resulted in increasing eating disorders in urban China (Yang 2011b).[6] Trying to achieve a thin body or face can be carried to an extreme that results in mental illness; however, the stigma associated with mental illness leads many Chinese with eating disorders to postpone treatment for as long as possible. When they do go, as mentioned, few doctors are trained to treat their condition.

Like other phenomena discussed in this chapter, disordered eating also has a class profile. Those who develop eating disorders tend to live a relatively comfortable lifestyle in urban environments, have good education, and be female (Björkell 2011). One 1999 study on disordered eating attitudes and behaviors compared high school girls in urban Hong Kong and similar samples of girls residing in two locations within Mainland China: largely rural Hunan Province and Shenzhen, a semi-urban, rapidly growing industrial center. The level of industrialization was found to mediate disordered eating attitudes and behaviors, such that girls in Hong Kong displayed the most pronounced eating disturbances and body dissatisfaction, followed, respectively, by girls in Shenzhen and Hunan Province (Lee and Lee 2000). Such differences may derive from rural attitudes that value physical strength and robust figures that allow women to successfully undertake agricultural activities, as opposed to an aesthetic of female thinness; the more traditional values may have a protective effect against eating disorders.

The ideological shift to naturalizing biological differences between men and women in the post-Mao reform era is a social construct defining the way men and women lead their lives, relate to each other, and access resources. Eating disorders in China are both effects of and contributors to this gender ideology shift that benefits men in satisfying their masculine gaze and masculine taste and meeting their preferences for a "weak" wife. It also benefits the state by implicitly facilitating state-led economic restructuring that requires women to return home owing to gendered layoffs.

## CONCLUSION

This chapter has explored the role of gender in the etiology, treatment, and management of mental distress. I have looked closely at the socially constructed differences between women and men in terms of roles and responsibilities, status and power, and at how these interact with biological differences between the sexes. I have queried how the social and the biological contribute to differences in the nature of mental health problems, health-seeking behaviors, and responses of the health sector and society. Gender-related experiences and stereotypes on the part of the psychiatrist may also influence diagnoses of depression and the higher rates of prescription of psychopharmaceutical drugs to women. While I have focused on gender-based epidemiological differences in depression and eating disorders in China, major gaps in our knowledge of other types of mental distress remain. We know more about the differences between males and females with regard to some mental health problems, like depression and schizophrenia, rather than others, and we know more about adult men and women than about adolescents and children. Gender stereotyping may also lead to under-diagnosis of mental health problems in men and over-diagnosis in women.

Mental health policies and programs in China should incorporate an understanding of gender issues. These should be developed in consultation with a diverse range of women and men, including service users. Reforms should combine a social justice approach and a public health approach in order to improve primary prevention and address risk factors, many of which are gender-specific. This implies going beyond medicalizing distress. If gender discrimination, gender-based violence, and gender-role stereotyping underlie at least some part of distress, they must be addressed through legislation and specific policies, programs, and interventions.

This chapter offers a gendered account of the role of specific forms of oppression based on gender inequality and gender complementarity in mental illness, that is, socially induced mental distress in a time of severe socioeconomic-political change in China. The chapter leans more strongly on the societal or structural sources of mental illness by showing how women are disproportionately affected by socioeconomic processes. In addition, a class analysis shows that even though the incidence and forms of distress may vary across class lines, both men and women are affected by structural threats to their lives. The gendered perspectives here show the greater effect these socioeconomic forces have on women and the dynamics between men and women, between class and gender. The analysis shows that the emphasis on the psychologization of mental distress in China implicitly downplays socioeconomic causes of mental distress.

Combining a consideration of men's forms of distress with women's modes of distress within the same class and across class boundaries, I highlight some of the complementarity between men's and women's experiences of distress. For example, job burnout and several of the apparently desired traits of masculinity (e.g., emotionlessness) serve to create men with few emotional resources with which to show empathy. But empathy and emotional connections are exactly the characteristics in men that women seek in their husbands and sons to boost their own sense of security when they are in need of support. So socialized gender norms exacerbate one another as they intersect. Women needing to build relational selves within family communities meet men unable to participate because they suffer either from *xiangpi ren* or from the pressures of trying to be a "typical" stoic man. Men, perhaps needing feminine support at home, find themselves called upon to provide that support themselves instead if a wife is stricken with mental distress, something they are ill prepared to do, so their situations can spiral downward. Essentialized psychological discourse confines the discussion of gender predominantly in the realm of heterosexual relationships and the domestic sphere, while downplaying the fact that gender is central to China's post-socialist transformation, structuring society and the political economy as a basic principle.

# 4    Stigma and Control ───────────

Go see a psychotherapist!
*A folk saying to curse people as insane*

I don't want to take medication; once taking it, I'll be really depressed.
*A woman diagnosed with major depressive disorder*

One of my informants, a psychiatrist in Beijing named Li (BJ-2013-d6), used the example of one of his patients to illustrate the current stigma associated with mental distress in China. One day a middle-aged woman came to see him at his clinic, telling him her daughter was suffering from some form of mental illness; she expected Li to offer a prescription to treat her daughter. When Li asked why the daughter had not come in person, the woman replied that her daughter did not think she was ill and had refused. When Li explained that he needed to see the daughter, the woman showed him a photo of the young woman. The psychiatrist again emphasized the necessity of seeing her in person, but the woman just reiterated that he could see her in photos – she could bring more, including images of her daughter from childhood until the present. This anecdote, Li told me, showed the woman's reluctance to convince her daughter to attend a psychiatric evaluation or reveal her identity, and the lengths family members will go to in order to prevent publicly exhibiting the mental health issues of loved ones. This mother preferred to control the doctor's view of her daughter, rather than have her daughter admit to her suffering by revealing herself bodily to his clinical gaze. This stigma, Li argued, prevents people from seeking treatment and can have devastating consequences both for sufferers and for those surrounding them.

One recent example of the consequences of stigma associated with mental disorder was the sensational murder case of a student at Sichuan Normal University on April 15, 2016. The student was slashed over 50 times with a kitchen knife by his roommate, purportedly because the latter was disturbed by his singing. Later, the roommate's mother confessed that her son has suffered from depression and had attempted suicide several times since high school. She had not revealed her son's mental situation to the university for fear of possible stigma and discrimination against him, which she believed would result in fewer prospects for his education and work life. The tragedy might have been avoided with the awareness of the state of the student's mental health, and appropriate treatment and supervision.

Indeed, in China, mental patients' occasional disruption of the social order and their failure to act in ways that promote social harmony are considered serious transgressions of social norms (Gao and Phillips 2001; Phillips 2001). A 1999 study about attitudes toward the mentally ill in Beijing found that over 60 percent of 254 randomly selected community members believed that persons with severe mental illnesses should not be allowed to marry or have children, and about 40 percent believed that the mentally ill should not be allowed to live in the community, return to work, or attend university (Gao and Phillips 2001). These beliefs make it extremely difficult for persons who suffer from a serious mental illness to obtain a job or get married, so most patients remain dependent on family members for life. Family members often delay necessary treatment for fear of being stigmatized and frequently go to extreme lengths to prevent neighbors and other acquaintances from discovering the family secret (Kleinman 1986). In most cases, the secret eventually comes out, resulting in severe negative consequences for the individual and the family. According to studies undertaken in several locations in China in the 1990s, 84 percent of family members of those who suffer from schizophrenia reported that social stigma affected the lives of healthy family members (Gao and Phillips 2001).

Multiple definitions of stigma have been put forward in recent years. For Graham Thornicroft and colleagues (2007), "stigma" comprises three interweaving elements: problems of knowledge (ignorance), problems of attitudes (prejudice), and problems of behavior (discrimination). Meanwhile, Bruce Link and Jo Phelan address both the social and psychological aspects of stigma in their definition, which includes four components:

> In the first component, people distinguish and label human differences. In the second, dominant cultural beliefs link labeled persons to undesirable characteristics – to negative stereotypes. In the third, labeled persons are placed in distinct categories so as to accomplish some degree of separation of "us" from "them." In the fourth, labeled persons experience status loss and discrimination that leads to unequal outcomes. (Link and Phelan 2001: 367)

Stigma has both micro- and macro-social consequences. Link and Phelan assert that research on stigma has attended primarily to its perception by individuals and its consequences for micro-level interactions. But stigmatic markers can classify entire groups of individuals and can have systemic implications for both individuals and groups.

The stigma associated with mental illness is viewed by the World Health Organization as a global barrier to the provision of mental health care. From a clinical perspective, stigma and ensuing discrimination have negative effects on the severity of symptoms, willingness to seek help, treatment patterns, and clinical outcomes for the mentally ill (Yang et al. 2007). In general, stigma may have negative effects on the social functioning of people with mental illness and on their employment. Stigma constrains the development of mental health programs, with structural discrimination hindering policy making and limiting service and research investment (Kleinman 1986, 1995; Li et al. 2014).

Understanding people's subjective experiences of stigma informs us of what is at stake in their lived local worlds: that is, their everyday interpersonal transactions involving family members, partners, friends, and colleagues (Kleinman and Kleinman 1997). It is thus important to examine the nature, magnitude, and impact of Chinese patients' experience of stigma in their local worlds (Lee et al. 2005). However, Chinese society has often been said to privilege interpersonal bonding over individualism. Without accounts of personal experience we cannot fully understand stigma. Nor can stigma in China be understood without exploring its relation to cultural tradition and to the current trend of therapeutic governance.

Thus, I want to take a multifaceted approach to stigma. While highlighting how stigma leads to inequitable treatment of individuals, in this chapter I also want to consider stigma as a vehicle for informal social control. My analysis shows that stigma in China can be individually painful, as well as a mode of governing through media and governments, and even a strategy of contestation and resistance when, for example, individuals who suffer from mental illness and their families manipulate and optimize the illness and its stigma for their own benefit. I focus in particular on the stigma surrounding schizophrenia and depression. I treat stigma as a means of defining access to resources and a political process in which feelings, experiences, and identities are constructed, discriminated against, and contested, all in the unique context of Chinese history and culture, and in relation to longstanding ideas about relationality and the self.

I contend that one of the key features of therapeutic governing of mental health in China is the use of stigma to control and regulate those who are afflicted. Stigmatic governance involves the use of "scientific" facts, shaming strategies, or simplistic or overly reductive models for categorizing or regulating social and political deviance. Stigmatic governing constructs subjects who are both vulnerable and strategic, subjected to but also optimizing stigma for their own advantages. Since culture and social context shape the expression, recognition, and social acceptance of psychiatric illnesses as well as the definition of stigma and the way people cope with it (Kleinman 1986), I will first contextualize the study of stigma associated with mental distress in the Chinese context and the Chinese notion of "face."

## STIGMA AND "FACE" IN CHINA

Most theoretical models define stigma psychologically and focus on its negative effects on individuals (Corrigan and Watson 2002). However, while acknowledging key roles that psychological forces play in stigma's manifestation in Western countries, scholars studying stigma in China note something different: the moral-somatic process of stigma, which affects both individuals and families (Kleinman 1986, 1995; Yang et al. 2007).[1] They propose that "face," as a distinctive cultural and moral phenomenon in China, plays an important role in the stigmatization process (Yang et al. 2007). Lawrence Hsin Yang and Arthur Kleinman (2008) offer a model highlighting how changes in moral status affect the functioning of stigma. They analyze how stigmas interact with social exchange networks that are organized based on reciprocal favors, moral positioning, and "face." The Chinese notion of "face" is primarily a moral category (*lian*), acting like an assessment of one's moral character and moral standing in a social context. It has another meaning too: public or social "face" (*mianzi*). Face, according to Yang and Kleinman (2008), is a physical, emotional, social, and moral process in Chinese society, which functions as a form of symbolic social capital analogous to *guanxi* (social ties) – a platform for economic, political, social, and recreational activities (Yan 1996). Through cultivating and maintaining one's moral face (*lian*), a person is able to obtain social face (*mianzi*), which influences the overall social capital and resources the person possesses (Yang and Kleinman 2008).

Despite having varied characteristics, the Chinese concept of "face" has its roots in Confucianism, which focuses on social harmony, stability, and hierarchy. Even today, people still consider it a great virtue and achievement for individuals to maintain harmonious relationships, especially with superiors, but also with peers and those who are lower in rank; achieving these goals is a way for people to obtain respect and unlock resources (Yang and Kleinman 2008). Conversely, mental illness precludes effective social networking. As a community-orientated society, China takes "face" as central to social identity; mental illness means being faceless or shamed (L.H. Yang 2007). To be mentally unfit and disruptive is to lose face. Chinese people tend to believe that, in such cases, ethical failure or moral lapses are at stake (partly because Confucianism values agency, action, or behavior more than thinking). Extending the prejudice of stigma to the family members of the mentally ill in China threatens to break social networks that might have linked these family members to social others, working opportunities, and additional social and capital resources (Yang and Kleinman 2008).

Jinhua Guo (2016) contends that in China stigma did not attract much public attention until the Chinese government defined the HIV/AIDS epidemic in the 1980s, which forced the country finally to start paying attention to the concept. As HIV/AIDS stigma has been increasingly recognized, both mass media and academic discourses have tended to attribute stigma to traditional cultural constructions, lack of knowledge, and lack of sympathy owing to the current social transformations and market competition (Guo 2016: 8). Stigma can be perpetuated through conscious or unconscious processes. Expressions of stigma can emerge within a family, or in a community, or in biases that come from service providers. Biases reinforce anger, fear, and prejudice.

Indeed, unlike typical expressions of stigma in the West reflecting a moral judgment of individuals, in China moral blame is applied to both individuals and their entire families (Kleinman 1995). Given fears about the potentially disruptive effects of mental illness, approaches to treating it often focus on control and only secondarily on treatment (Kleinman 1995). Stigma is attached not only to mental illness but also to the spaces and professionals of mental health treatment. *Qu kan kan xinli yisheng ba* (Go to see a psychotherapist) used to be a way of cursing people who were viewed as insane or "out of their minds" in the 1990s. A doctor of internal medicine at the same hospital in which the mental health center ZYH is located often heard people caution him to take particular care of himself when he first started working there several years ago. The town where ZYH is located is even somewhat stigmatized; one of the psychiatrists at ZYH decided to move his family out of the community close to the hospital because of his son constantly complaining about his classmates ridiculing him for living in *that* crazy community.

## STIGMA AGAINST SCHIZOPHRENIA

Schizophrenia offers a strong test case of stigma in China. Its place as a psychiatric disorder is far different than that of, for example, depression (see below). In China (and in the West), schizophrenia frequently appears in media representations, including film, as the ultimate sickness, or even as a mark of genius. In part, this is because this illness category remains mysterious. As Michael Green has argued: "Schizophrenia is shrouded in an overpowering sense of mystery. … When an illness is viewed as inexplicable and impenetrable, people tend to react to it with one of the two extremes: either they *stigmatize* the illness or they *romanticize* it" (2003: 1, italics in the original). In China, *jingshen fenlie* (schizophrenia) is more stigmatized than romanticized. The media associate schizophrenia with violence, which criminalizes those who have developed the disorder. Public education about the biology of schizophrenia – as an illness of the brain for which no one is at fault – attempts to offset widespread stigma associated with the label and reinforce existing biomedical treatments. Brain disease in China represents something seemingly more complicated and harder to treat than psychological issues. This may be why one man I met at MKH in summer 2013, who had recovered from schizophrenia, nonetheless stayed in hospital. He told me that he had nowhere to go. Neither his family nor his original community wanted to take him back because of the strong stigma against schizophrenia and the association of the condition with violence, disruption, and untreatability.

Another of my informants in Zhangqiu named Sun (ZYH-2015-p6), described how, upon returning home from work one day, she saw her husband Zhang Jilin, who has suffered from schizophrenia for over 35 years, surrounded by a group of men. Zhang was naked, performing a handstand against the wall while the villagers laughed and cheered him on. Sun was enraged. She yelled at them, "Are you human? Don't you know he is sick? Are you all sick!? Good people don't do things like this, bullying someone who has suffered so much. He used to be as healthy as you are and make much more money than any of you can make but got sick because of a job injury, nothing else, okay?" For Sun, to restore her husband's and her own family's reputation required this move to let people know Zhang's history, the before-and-after of his job injury – a way of restoring his face, and the face and dignity of his family. (Zhang was traumatized in a coal mining accident and subsequently developed symptoms of schizophrenia – see Chapter 5.) Sun pulled off her coat, covered her husband's body, and took him home – the fourth place to which she had moved since the onset of his illness. Owing to the stigma and discrimination against her husband and son, she has moved from village to village. Because of her husband's illness, her son had difficulty finding a marriage partner. Finally, when he was in his late thirties, Sun helped him find a wife.

She did not want the stigma to ruin the marriage. But there seems to be no place where they (the son lives with his parents) can live respectably and "normally." Indeed, in the above-mentioned 1999 survey about attitudes toward mental illness in Beijing, over 40 percent of the 211 patients with schizophrenia interviewed felt that their work unit discriminated against them and that neighbors looked down on them and their family; 28 percent reported moving to avoid stigma (Gao and Phillips 2001).

According to Sun, the stigma resulting from her husband's illness can be subtle. At the third village they moved to, one of her neighbors came to complain that Zhang's singing of Beijing opera at home was so loud that it was making their dog bark. The barking often awakened this neighbor's newborn daughter. Sun replied that it might be easier and more appropriate to control a dog than a sick man whose only entertainment as a human being is singing Beijing opera. But she soon figured out that the neighbor had more in mind than Zhang's singing. Sun was not surprised when, a few days later, her landlord asked them to move, saying he had received complaints from neighbors and warnings from the village committee. In this case, stigma became a form of regulation and a mode of governing at the grassroots level. During the last 35 years of taking care of her husband, Sun complained that none of the village committees had ever offered any help or poverty relief, but rather had sidelined or even ignored her small family in various poverty relief programs, partly because of stigma and the popular association between schizophrenia and violence.

However, Sun could also be strategic about unfair treatment. Whenever conflict arose or the family was mistreated by village committees, she involved her husband as a means of making her situation more public. Zhang would curse them, making a scene by revealing the committee's wrongs, and "reasoning" with them, which sometimes worked in the family's favor. For example, when the family was ignored during Chinese New Year, when "households in particular difficulty" (*tekunhu*) should receive *song wenuan*, or "sending warmth," Zhang's persistence led to a symbolic gift: a bag of flour and a bottle of cooking oil (see Yang 2013). Then Sun would explain to people bothered by her husband that those who suffer schizophrenia do not distinguish good from bad, and do not know how to stop cursing. In such cases, Sun used the idea of mental illness as contagion against those who had offended and marginalized her. She would send the contagious person – her husband Zhang – into the spaces of her "enemies," who would be forced to deal with him at close range, and also hear, publicly, about their own bad deeds. Sun's redeployment of stigma went beyond strategy to become a mode of defense and a political tool.

If Sun's case shows how stigma can be circulated and even used as self-defense, in other cases stigma is used to negotiate major systems – like the medical system – as well as to exert social control over family members. Perceptions of stigma can affect the choice of psychiatrists and treatment patterns. One of my informants named Lili (MKH-2015-p6), whom I met at Beijing MKH, was diagnosed with schizophrenia during a period when she was looking for work. During the first five years of her diagnosis, she was unable to find a psychiatrist whose treatments stabilized her condition. Her parents finally found a psychiatrist at MKH. This psychiatrist, Dr. Yuan, was well known for being "heavy-handed," prescribing much bigger doses of psychopharmaceuticals than other psychiatrists, which were often efficacious, but with harmful side-effects. Lili's parents struggled: while they did not want their daughter to suffer from crippling side-effects, they were eager to get her symptoms under control. During that period, at night Lili often cried, screamed, and kicked her parents' bedroom door. Although they had tried hard to make their apartment soundproof, they were concerned that neighbors and colleagues would discover their daughter's mental distress, which would harm her and negatively impact their own job prospects. In the end, they decided to try Dr. Yuan's prescription, and Lili's symptoms did come under control. She was able to find a job. With this employment prospect, Lili's parents have started to work hard to find her a husband and secure a "normal" life for her. In her early thirties, Lili is already perceived as a "leftover woman" (*shengnv*). Worse yet, of five boyfriends, none would continue to see her after she told them the history of her schizophrenia and about the medication she takes – a small dose now, but one necessary to maintain her mental equilibrium.

Lili's parents worry about her marriage prospects, as she is getting older. They have since consulted different psychiatrists, searching for one who would tell them when their daughter could finally stop taking anti-psychotics. They also wonder about her future. If Lili finally gets married and becomes pregnant, could she stop medication to avoid negative effects on the fetus, but still maintain her own health? Their mission now is to sort out all these issues so they can convince other boyfriends that their daughter is safe to date. Lili appears to have little control over her body, which in many ways belongs to her parents as well. Indeed, health is both a personal and a family affair in China (see Chapter 1). Families want desperately to align their ill loved ones with convention in order to save them from being abandoned, but also to save themselves. Stigma therefore encourages a kind of physical surveillance of the ill person to the point of guiding their marriage and reproductive lives, as in the case of Lili and her parents.

As reproductive health is central to social reproduction, efforts to avoid detection of mental illness during one's reproductive years seem especially great. Another informant of mine, who suffers from schizophrenia but whose symptoms are controlled, got married without revealing her medical history or medication to her husband. After she got pregnant, she stopped taking medication to avoid possible negative effects on the fetus. Unfortunately, she soon manifested symptoms of schizophrenia, including hallucination, altered speech styles, and behaviors that bewildered her husband and his family. Finally, she had to tell them the truth. Her husband was at first shocked and enraged but reconciled with her because of the baby they were going to have. In this situation, the unborn baby became the excuse for the couple to stay together. China's collectivist culture does not protect psychiatric patients against familial stigma; stigma can lead to breaks with even the closest people in one's life. Intrafamilial and social connections can break down in the face of the powerful forces of stigma (Kleinman and Kleinman 1997). Studies in China indicate that families might ultimately abandon a member with schizophrenia. Such abandonment is particularly distressing because unmarried adults are generally expected to live with their parents and siblings. Abandoned family members can therefore be left literally without social resources (Lee 2002).

The degree of negative attitudes toward people with schizophrenia is higher than it is toward those with depression. Studying the incentive effects of stigma, Lawrence Blume (2002) suggests that the cost of being stigmatized is low when many people bear the marker, and highest when only a few are thus marked. Indeed, depression has now become one of the most widespread forms of mental distress in China. Many more people bear the marker (about 11 percent) than in the case of schizophrenia (about 1 percent). In addition, people are more inclined to attribute depression to stress, which they do not do with schizophrenia (Li et al. 2014). One of my informants named Leng, from Zhangqiu, was originally diagnosed as schizophrenic at ZYH (ZYH-2015-p16). Later, fearing discrimination by her colleagues and employer, Leng, who had recently given birth, switched to a well-known mental hospital in Beijing, where she described typical symptoms of postpartum depression to the psychiatrist (about 80 percent of new mothers experience some degree of anxiety and depression after giving birth in China[2]). She had familiarized herself with these symptoms online before her visit. While someone suffering from schizophrenia could have symptoms that overlapped with these, Leng put them in the context of her status as a new mother, and the psychiatrist duly diagnosed her with postpartum depression. This allowed her to obtain extra sick leave, with less stigma and discrimination from her employer. However, to contain her symptoms, Leng continued to see psychiatrists at ZYH, whom she had visited for years. She was also occasionally hospitalized and treated as someone with schizophrenia. Leng's move to recast her symptoms as postpartum depression leaves open the likelihood that they are stress induced, which schizophrenia is putatively not, and evidences the importance of reproductive issues in Chinese society – resulting in a lower stigma associated with post-partum depression (as well as other forms of depression) than that associated with schizophrenia.

## STIGMA AGAINST DEPRESSION

In China, estimates are that about 90 million people suffer from depression (Gao and Liu 2016). Every year 200,000 people commit suicide because of depression (Gao and Liu 2016). The antidepressant market is booming, while health services struggle to cope with the numbers in need of treatment. The illness is generally viewed in Chinese society as a result of weak will or weak personality. Owing to such stigma and overall misassumptions, only 4 percent of those who suffer depression are treated (Zhang Jin 2016). Yet about 80 percent of those sufferers admitted to hospitals can recover, and of those, 20 percent show no signs of relapse (Zhang Jin 2016). As mentioned in Chapter 1, in Chinese, *yiyu* (depression) has multivalent and diverse meanings and connotations. *Yiyu* in general refers to both a heart-emotion (or depressive state) and an illness category (major depressive disorder), which is more stable and long-lasting. We can thus understand depressive symptoms to be indicative either of individual disease, caused by personal biology or biography, or an illness of distress, caused by conditions outside the person, including sociopolitical-economic pressures – or both.

How depression is perceived influences treatment. One perspective is that depression can be resolved with *xiangkai* (thinking out): if one opens one's heart, behaves and acts happily and is social, one will feel better. According to one online poll, 88.7 percent of Chinese believe that depression can be cured through *ziwo tiaojie* (self-adjustment) or *xiangkai* without professional medical treatment.[3] The other perspective is that depression is a condition analogous to breaking one's leg. Without seeing a doctor, one's broken leg will not heal. It will not recover just because one changes to a new environment, adopts a new heart-attitude, or becomes more social and meets new friends. However, most people in China do not have easy access to qualified specialists, especially outside cities such as Beijing and Shanghai. According to a 2009 survey by the Shanghai Mental Health Centre, between 2001 and 2005, 88 percent of China's patients with mental disorders did not receive any professional treatment (Kaiman 2013). Arguably, under-treating depression costs China in other ways: the illness results in approximately US$6.6 billion annually in lost workdays and other financial burdens (Kaiman 2013).

The diagnosis of depression is included in the *Chinese Classification of Mental Disorders* (CCMD), with many similar criteria to the World Health Organization's *International Classification of Diseases* (ICD) or the American Psychiatric Association's *Diagnostic and Statistical Manual of Mental Disorders* (DSM). However, neurasthenia was once a more prominent diagnosis, particularly in the 1980s (Kleinman 1986). Although also found in the *ICD*, its diagnosis takes a particular form in China, called *shenjing shuairuo* (literally translated as "weak neurology"), which emphasizes somatic complaints as well as fatigue or depressed feelings. Neurasthenia is a less stigmatizing diagnosis than depression in China, being conceptually distinct from psychiatric labels and said to fit well with a tendency to express emotional issues in somatic terms, therefore it was culturally and politically appropriate in the 1980s (Kleinman 1995). The concept of neurasthenia as a nervous system disorder is also perceived to suit the traditional Chinese epistemology of disease causation on the basis of disharmony of vital organs and imbalance of $qi$ (life force; see Chen 2003; Lee 2011). However, neurasthenia has recently been replaced as the primary clinical diagnosis in China and depression has become the new "normal."

Many people in China try their best to hide symptoms of depression with smiling faces. They act "normal" or "positive" without acknowledging the seriousness of their condition. They believe that if they continue acting "normal," their depression will disappear on its own. Culturally, people are socialized to hide "black holes" in their emotional lives. That is, people believe they should not reveal their depression or turn their emotions into negative energy, spreading them among friends and then becoming other people's burden. One should care about "face" in order to sustain social harmony and collective solidarity (see Yang and Kleinman 2008). To destigmatize depression, it is important to understand it in its multiplicity as a heart-emotion, as subjective experience, and as a set of brain disorders. Some of my informants indicated that depression is a devil, destroying their lives. Others depicted it as an accompanying "black dog" which ruins one's appetite and eats one's ability to memorize and to concentrate; one nevertheless has to carry it with extraordinary perseverance. Still others said that depression is a test, a miraculous design by God for those who suffer depression to figure out what death means and how to live.

Owing to the persistent stigma attached to mental disorders in China, people deploy various strategies to show others that they are not marked with/by such disorders, for example by invoking physical illness or other less stigmatized idioms of distress (Nichter 2010). One of my informants, named Huo (MKH-2012-p3), whom I met at MKH, had gone there seeking treatment for "menopause syndrome," which included low spirits, exhaustion, and loss of interest in almost everything, lying in bed all day without motivation or energy to do anything. But when the doctor checked her personal information, she was only 42 and had no sign of approaching menopause at all. The doctor diagnosed her as suffering from medium to severe depression. While Huo did not dispute the diagnosis, she asked the doctor to write her medical record in terms of symptoms, without directly mentioning the term "depression," so that she could ask for sick leave from her employer based on menopause syndrome, rather than the more stigmatized depression. As a director of a bank branch, she indicated that she had to be very cautious to represent herself as not associated in any way with serious illness, especially mental illness, which would stigmatize her as impotent, weak, and lacking rationality. In her view, health itself contains an element of primary power, providing control over her body and lifestyle. That is, if one is not healthy, one's ability to manage one's body and daily life is placed in doubt. Illnesses bring with them the stigma of impotence and paralyze one's autonomy and social prestige, while enhancing one's dependence on other healthy people. From this perspective, health is control; illness breaches authority. Huo contended that (mental) health is necessary for the possession of social and political power. Stigma against mental illness in this case encompasses a socioeconomic, somatic, and intersubjective process that frames and legitimizes one's relationship to others and one's social and economic status.

*Officials' depression and suicide: stigma and self-stigma*

Many Chinese go to extreme lengths to avoid the stigma of mental illness. Besides making efforts to hide symptoms of distress, they also use cultural idioms that somatize mental distress, as in the case of Huo, or the way neurasthenia has been used in China. Owing to fear of discrimination and self-stigmatization, some Chinese officials I interviewed took measures to hide their "depression" from employers and colleagues (see Chapter 1). Chinese bureaucratic culture creates high levels of self-stigma that lead to distorted self-images, isolation, and inconsistent diagnosis and treatment. Meanwhile, official media reinforce the stigma attached to mental illness, which further controls individuals and downplays the sociopolitical factors contributing to officials' mental disorders. However, officials sometimes also manipulate the stigma of depression to their own advantage.

Patrick Corrigan and Amy Watson (2002) point out that stigmatization has two dimensions: public stigma, which encompasses the reaction of the general population to people exhibiting mental distress, and self-stigma, which is the prejudice people exhibiting this distress turn against themselves. Public and self-stigma are often interrelated; both can constitute modes of control. For example, Arthur Kleinman (1995) argues that Chinese society's concern with social control intensifies the stigmatic effects of epilepsy. In this sense, stigma is the vehicle used for social control. To avoid stigma, families conceal diagnoses and sequester epileptic members at home. Likewise, many officials, who experience complicated emotions at work as a result of pressures to conform and fear of public condemnation, take various measures to hide their mental distress from employers and colleagues. Some in Zhangqiu secretly visit folk healers for psychological relief. Meanwhile, their problems continue to worsen.

Self-stigma can lead to isolation, lower self-esteem, and a distorted self-image (Kleinman 1995; Corrigan and Watson 2002). The stigma of having a mental illness is one of the most significant obstacles preventing Chinese officials from seeking help. A psychiatrist at MKH commented on the role of public stigma and self-stigma in depression.

They [officials] often think they are part of an elite group – the solution not the problem – and equate depression with weak will and incapability. … A senior provincial official came to me from Hebei Province and insisted that he didn't feel depressed; depression for him was a sign of weakness. He only suffered from insomnia and headaches. He refused to take any medicine for depression and his wife begged me to instead write that all the anti-depression medicine was for insomnia or headaches so that he might take it.

Given the extensive public stigma against those who show symptoms of mental illness or distress, people internalize the social ethos. When experiencing symptoms of mental distress, they actually stigmatize themselves. This adds self-pressure to social pressure to conceal one's symptoms. For Chinese officials, the resulting pressure can be tremendous, as they seek to avoid revealing any signs of distress so as not to negatively influence already competitive bureaucratic processes, such as promotion, that affect their lives. Indeed, competition among officials is stiff, which makes them feel helpless and closes off channels for communication and catharsis. If they are always worried that their rivals might recognize their weakness or mental illness in daily interactions, they experience extreme psychological pressure to conceal their symptoms.

One of my informants, an official from the local environmental preservation bureau in Zhangqiu, asked me to refer him to a psychiatrist by first telling me that his cousin had symptoms of bipolar disorder. Two years later, he revealed to me that it was he himself who suffered from this condition. He hoped to get it under control, as he was in line to be promoted to the position of department chief. As he was facing tense competition from his rivals, disclosure of his mental illness would mean career suicide. Similarly, a psychiatrist in Beijing indicated that through conversation with one of his patients, a woman in her seventies, he discovered that she was borrowing symptoms to get a diagnosis and prescription for her son, rather than herself. When the psychiatrist asked her to describe detailed subjective experiences of her depression, she simply could not, revealing her ruse. Her son, a powerful senior municipal official, had decided it was too risky to jeopardize his reputation and career prospects by exposing his mental distress. These examples illustrate the intertwining of public and private stigmatization and its possible social and political implications for those who suffer from mental distress (and for their families).

Given the role of stigma in enhancing patients' anxiety and the pressure they feel, psychiatrists with whom I spoke in Beijing indicated that they do not ask about clients' identities or positions if it is irrelevant to their mental health. Having their psychiatrist know of their public responsibilities only creates additional pressure and exacerbates their mental distress. One of the psychiatrists at ZYH, Dr. Li (ZYH-2015-d7), stated:

> Officials can easily tell people that they suffer high blood pressure but never reveal that they are suffering cancer or depression. The moment someone tells colleagues he has cancer, he is politically dead. If he reveals that he is suffering from depression, people render whatever he did or will do illegitimate, seeing all his behaviors as insane. He loses his credibility. … Leaders seldom go to a mental hospital by themselves. They usually ask their secretary to invite me [to join them] for meals. I, of course, know a leader's illness is top secret. When I bump into some of my patients on the street, I always try my best to avoid them. If I greet them, those who accompany them would wonder why they know a psychiatrist, which may embarrass them or intensify their pressure.

In Dr. Li's view, self-stigma depends on social stigma. He argues that a blend of social stigma and self-reproach can ultimately slow down treatment of mental illness and even intensify patients' experiences of social pressure as well as their symptoms. Afflicted individuals internalize the social prejudice and so turn their feelings of prejudice toward mental illness against themselves.

Some people afflicted with distress, however, manipulate the diagnosis of mental illness for their own advantage. A deputy director at the transportation bureau in Zhangqiu tried to leave the public sector to become a lawyer because of his constant failure to get promoted and his resentment of "hidden rules" (see Chapter 1) and demotion in his workplace. His efforts to secure a six-month leave to prepare for his bar examination were unsuccessful. Finally he went to the local hospital and told them he suffered insomnia, anxiety, and depression. With his diagnosis of depression in hand, he obtained his leave and is now a successful lawyer. He manipulated his symptoms in order to get the diagnosis of depression, which many still often attribute to environmental factors. He deliberately chose depression over, for example, schizophrenia, as the latter has greater stigma attached to it, and is held to be incurable, which would thereby impact his future practice as a lawyer. Also it is harder to manipulate the symptoms of schizophrenia, especially when, as was the case with this man, people do not know what these symptoms are. It is much easier to imitate the symptoms of depression, as it has become as widespread and popular as the flu. Much to this man's surprise, the diagnostic procedures were also quite "easy." The doctor wrote the diagnosis without even asking him why he could not sleep, or what other symptoms he might have. Within five minutes he had been sent to the hospital's pharmacy. This man's remarks also reveal how the diagnostic procedures assume a biomedical basis in the individual, which may contribute to the widespread biomedical perception of "depression" in China. The complexities of situational depression (associated with social and environmental factors) and biomedically induced depression are to the fore here. But because many others (especially medical professionals) think of depression as primarily biomedical, this official succeeded in getting a diagnosis and prescription without difficulty.

*Stigma against psychopharmaceutical drugs*

One of the stigmas or misperceptions about depression as both a heart-emotion and an illness category is that one can recover if one keeps being positive and socially engaged by readjusting oneself and exercising. Once taking medication, it is argued, one will get addicted and then will become really sick. One day, I received a text message from an outpatient I met at ZYH, a woman in her mid-thirties, asking me to convince her mother not to make her take medication. When I called, she told me that her mother had threatened to put her in the mental hospital if she continued to refuse to take the prescribed drugs. For this woman, taking drugs meant she would not be able to use her willpower and self-adjustment through her meditation and yoga practices to redress her depressive mood, and her condition would develop into depression as a disease. She further believed that drugs would make her feel worse. Having read closely about the function and possible side-effects of these drugs in the manuals, she anticipated becoming a psychiatric patient once she started to take them. Indeed, many in China still have a strong sense of stigma associated with psychopharmaceutical drugs.

As a response to such popular "misconceptions," a widely circulating public discourse permeating Chinese media has vehemently criticized those who suffer from severe depression but refuse to take medication, and has even condemned those who refuse professional medical assistance as "animals" who do not know how to use the "tools" of biomedical treatment and drugs. From this perspective, enduring the pain and suffering caused by symptoms of severe depression is a sign of foolishness and primitiveness. This discourse downplays the agency of those who suffer severe depression to choose their own path to healing, whether that path is social, physical, medical, or some combination of these resources. Instead, this discourse highlights the efficacy of psychopharmaceutical drugs, implicitly advancing the pharmaceutical industry.[4]

The media and the government advocate for a biomedical definition of depression as a disease (see Chapter 1 on the discussion of "officials' heartache"). Yet many of my informants, while suffering from medium to severe depression, refuse drug treatment, hoping they will recover through self-adjustment, exercise, and other alternative healing systems (also see Chapter 1). Indeed, for many, depression is multivalent, and its treatment diverse. Treatment can also include counseling and Chinese herbal medicine – the latter as a means of evading stigma and side-effects. As noted, many associate psychopharmaceutical drugs with addiction. They believe that starting a drug regimen will plunge them into real depression and get them addicted. Despite assurances from psychiatrists, patients remain unconvinced, partly owing to the biomedical jargon in which abstract explanations are offered. I did hear once a very clear explanation of drug use during my field research in Beijing. Dr. Lan (MKH-2012-d9) used a metaphor: someone breaks her leg and needs crutches to walk. The crutch is the drugs. She cannot immediately abandon the crutches once she feels better. It will take time to fully recover and gradually stop relying on the crutches. Otherwise, she will fall again and get worse. Similarly, it takes time to stop taking antidepressant drugs in order to avoid withdrawal symptoms.

## STIGMA, CONTROL, AND TREATMENT

Social control can be exercised through invoking stigma or labels to demonize or criminalize those who suffer from mental distress. With the purported goal of further regulating and "caring" for those who suffer from mental illness, the Public Health and Family Planning Bureau of Shuangliu District, Chengdou, Sichuan Province, recently offered, via its official microblog, a reward of 350 yuan to anyone who identified and reported suspected psychiatric sufferers (Yu 2016). This type of reward- or tip-driven mass mobilization has often been applied in China to ferret out people engaging in illicit acts, such as criminals, corrupt officials, or drug dealers. It is telling, therefore, that the word *jubao*, which is linked to reporting criminal or corrupt activity, is used in this context. People are encouraged to "offer tip-offs" by identifying those who suffer from psychiatric diseases, thereby implicitly treating the latter as guilty of wrongdoing. To avoid being reported this way, it is likely that those who suffer psychiatric diseases will hide them all the more strenuously. Indeed, the Mental Health Law indicates that psychiatric patients who may potentially pose a serious risk of harming others can be forcibly hospitalized. Prevention of violence, however, should remain separate from questions of mental distress and its stigmatization, since usually the latter has nothing to do with violence (see Yu 2016).

Yet China's community-based mental health system focuses on controlling and treating psychoses, especially those associated with violent or socially disruptive behaviors. In September 2004, mental health was officially included in public health in China (Liu et al. 2011). The mental health reform program formally received support from the Ministry of Finance in December 2004, and was named the 686 Program after its initial funding of CNY6.86 million. According to Liu and colleagues (2011), by early 2005, 60 model sites were established, with one urban and one rural area in each of the 30 provinces of China, covering a population of 43 million. The priority in the first year was to build a capable mental health workforce through an extensive training program. In 2006, the 686 Program incorporated an intervention component into the training program. Four types of psychoses were included: schizophrenia, bipolar disorder, delusional disorder, and schizoaffective disorder (Liu et al. 2011: 212). Sufferers screened for possible psychosis were examined by psychiatrists, and those who met diagnostic criteria for psychotic disorders were evaluated for their risk of violence based on a 0 to 5 scale established by the national working group. Patients at risk of violence received a monthly followup and, if they were socioeconomically disadvantaged, were provided with free medication, laboratory tests, and a subsidy for hospitalization (Liu et al. 2011: 212).

From the social stability point of view, it is easy to understand why psychosis treatment and management is the top priority of the government. Owing to inefficient implementation of the new Mental Health Law, involuntary admission is undertaken under the name of "caring for the mentally ill" (Liu et al. 2011) – a form of kindly therapeutic governance. While such community-based mental health interventions partly alleviate the mental health "crisis," given the stigma against mental patients among community health care workers (see Li et al. 2014), stigma against mental distress has not entirely lifted. In fact, the attention to violence associated with severe psychoses in these recent mental health programs tends to increase popular stigmatization of all mental illnesses. When those who suffer severe psychotic disorders are selected for "treatment" by community mental health programs based on a potential for violence, public awareness of the association of mental illness with violence results in increased stigma and a more general bias. This pressures people to hide their mental distress. To lift the stigma of mental illness will require systematic social, economic, and political change that prioritizes quality psychiatric treatment, mental health care, and socioeconomic empowerment than top-down control and the emphasis on violent predilections.

## CONCLUSION

This chapter has explored how stigma in China is at once an intersubjective and intrasubjective experience that causes difficulties for individuals with mental illness and serves as a means of social control. Stigma is a kind of dialectic that exists between the state and the populace; as long as the state pursues therapeutic governance in ways that promote ignorance, stigma will be a tool for social control. The state has therefore provoked a situation in which people are not only subject to stigma (pain and suffering), but also use it pragmatically to unlock resources for themselves (e.g., in the strategic stigmatization of officials' depression).

Since stigma may build up over time, opportune intervention is required to turn families into long-term resources for psychiatric care (Lee 2002); this might, in turn, buffer patients and their caregivers against stigma in the public domain. I have given examples of families hiding mentally ill members and, presumably, taking responsibility for their care. The home constitutes a more positive, productive, and helpful form of mental health care in China. Given the large number of patients with chronic mental disorders in the country, community and home-based care for most patients is a realistic means of support. However, development of efficient and humanitarian community-based mental health care also requires careful attention; such programs can be problematic if they act as mechanisms of informal social control of "deviance" that reinforce stigma against mental distress and imprison sufferers of mental symptoms within a realm of prejudice shared between the public and themselves.

Overcoming stigma is difficult and challenging. As a tool of social control, it can be mismanaged, reinforced, or dispelled. A biological explanation of mental illness disseminated by Chinese media and government may help to dispel some of the stigma of guilt and shame, particularly when the patient and family understand that mental illnesses such as schizophrenia are related to biological neurotransmitter imbalances. However, such biologization can reinforce mental illness as only a personal or biological matter, downplaying social factors contributing to social distress and intensifying control over individuals. Lawrence Hsin Yang and Arthur Kleinman (2008: 12) propose to combat stigmatization via the restoration of "face" for individuals and families. They focus interventions on local contexts related to moral status, for example through "remoralization counseling."

This entails a complex of counseling for those afflicted with mental distress to counteract internalized stigma or self-stigma by replacing notions of moral deprecation with the belief that even those with chronic illnesses are capable of contributing productively to society.

This remoralization counseling involves coaching strategies to reach desired vocational and interpersonal outcomes (e.g., employment, dating) as well as nuanced strategies for "selectively disclosing" a stigmatized status to employers and potential romantic partners (Yang and Kleinman 2008: 12) However, the Chinese government has used stigma (or destigmatization) as a mode of governance, for example through psychologization within a bureaucratic order by labeling Chinese officials' suicides as due to the individual illness of biomedical depression. Therefore, a combination of micro- and macro-level intervention (intersubjective interaction, government-sponsored media educational campaigns, and policies of destigmatization) will be essential in destigmatizing mental illness in China. In general, this analysis of stigma offers a framework that explores Chinese ways of thinking about the body, medicine, morality, subjectivity, family, and the state.

# 5 Psychopharmacology, Subjectivity, and Psychiatric Hospital Care

On March 10, 2009, a division director of Beijing Huairou Anjia Hospital, Dr. Yang, was killed by a mental patient in the process of discharging him. This is the first reported killing of a psychiatrist by a mental patient in Beijing.

On June 16, 2014, a man suffering from schizophrenia ran away from Shandong Guangji Psychiatric Hospital, killing one care worker and injuring two more when they tried to retrieve him.

On May 5, 2016, Dr. Chen Zhongwei of Guangdong People's Hospital was killed at home by a man diagnosed as psychotic.

Recent years have witnessed a series of such events taking place in and around Chinese hospitals that treat mental illness. I present these events not to imply that mental health issues are correlated with violence (they are not), nor to echo media narratives about "crazy" individuals as the cause of social unrest (in China this has more to do with socioeconomic dislocation). Rather, I contend that such events illustrate the problems of China's mental health care system, which relate to privatization and to the dominant treatment model, which emphasizes the use of psychiatric drugs not just to aid people's rapid recovery, but also to reduce possibly violent behaviors. Paradoxically, recent violent events can also be interpreted as social consequences of drug-based psychiatric treatment, which does not (fully) address social or psychological causes of mental illness. In this respect, while psychiatry as currently practiced in China mostly aligns with the aims of therapeutic governance – that is, to manage and regulate the population through psychological care – its control is incomplete, and has unintended consequences.

In my ethnographic research, I encountered cases that connected violence, the law, and psychiatric care. One such case is revealed by Dr. Ge, a psychiatrist at MKH (MKH-2013-d16). He tells of a woman who moved to his residential community several years ago. She refused to be confined to her home or receive medical treatment for distress, behaving in ways that her loved ones and community members viewed as a "relapse" of psychotic symptoms. She would constantly talk nonsense while throwing things from her fourth-floor apartment. She patrolled the community carrying a chef's knife, glaring at or attacking anyone who looked her way. She once used cobblestones to attack neighbors. Residents called the local police, who in turn sent her to the local mental hospital, but she was released just days later. Under the 2013 Mental Health Law, without the agreement of her two brothers, who are her designated caretakers but live in another city, neither the residents' committee nor the police could do more than send her to hospital occasionally to be medicated. As mentioned in Chapter 4, given the public's fear of the mentally ill and their potentially disruptive effects, the community approach to mental illness in China is primarily focused on control and only secondarily on treatment (Kleinman 1986). In this case, the community did not seem to do either very efficiently. Many questions remain unanswered: What will become of this woman? If her violent behavior continues, what will the consequences be for her neighbors? If forcible confinement is barred, what other treatment will the government offer – for her and her community? More fundamentally, how do this woman and others who suffer from similar conditions, in and out of hospital, view themselves? Do their views change when they take medication versus when they do not? And how are they viewed by others – their doctors, the law, and their communities?

Underlying these questions is a deeper set of queries about the factors contributing to mental disorders, whether social or biological or both, and how they are treated. In his study of Romanian psychiatry, Jack Friedman (2016) argues that as social problems increasingly contribute to the suffering of those with mental distress, mental health care has become heavily focused on psychopharmacological treatment. Similarly, in China, psychiatric care at hospitals is predominantly psychopharmacological and this, in the context of widespread dislocation, cannot alleviate distress.

Treatment of severe mental illness in China, however, is unique in scope and response. About 10 percent of the 16 million Chinese with severe mental disorders reportedly show a tendency toward physical violence (Liu 2016). Because of limited social and medical resources, most of these people are literally locked at home without treatment. In Hebei Province alone, there are about 100,000 such "caged people" (*longzhong ren*) (Liu 2016). Through a project called *jie suo gongcheng* (unlocking programs), mental hospitals can take the initiative to bring back some of those people for medical treatment. However, because of the implementation of China's new Mental Health Law, which protects the privacy and freedom of patients and their guardians, the project of unlocking mental patients in Hebei Province has stalled (Liu 2016). For the majority of severely mentally ill patients, iron cages may indeed be their ultimate fate, owing to financial limitations, lack of family care, and fear within their communities.

In this chapter, I address this state of affairs and, in particular, the new forms of subjectivity arising within China's current mental health care approaches. I problematize the reductive psychopharmacological approaches dominating (though unevenly) hospital-based psychiatric practice in China. These therapies redraw the boundaries of subjectivity for people in mental distress through a biomedical approach that diminishes what João Biehl and colleagues (2007) would call the vital local, relational, and social aspects of the self. However, the reduction in subjective boundaries is never total. Rather, those with mental disorders are designated and re-designated: as biologically based individuals, as "sick," as beloved family members, as dangers to the community, as rights-bearing citizens under the law, as patients, as pet projects of caring doctors and nurses, and more. I contend that this uneven development of patient subjectivity offers room for mental patients and their family members to negotiate and contest the treatment they receive and its side-effects. Contrary to the biomedical conception of patients as primarily biochemical organisms, families often attempt to maintain a rich subjective experience for those on the drugs by keeping them engaged with life in general through personal care. Even nurses and doctors at times attempt to enlarge the subjectivity of patients through personal attention or occasional talk therapy, but they are ultimately bound to the dominant psychopharmacological model. In fact, personal care given at hospitals is typically viewed as facilitating psychopharmacological treatment. I pay particular attention to the body as a force combating side-effects of psychotic drugs and a key site for subject formation.

## PSYCHOPHARMACOLOGY AND SUBJECTIVITY

The notion of subjectivity that I pursue here is in line with what Biehl et al. (2007) propose: that is, the sense of one's self and one's place in the world. Subjectivity is multi-faceted and contextualized, including historically situated differences in social sensibility and what it means to feel and regard oneself as human. I explore subjectivities with consideration of cross-cultural differences in cognition, affect, and action. Culture shapes the behavioral environment and the selves who inhabit that environment, as well as the moods and motivations that are part of these selves (Biehl et al. 2007: 7). The subject is at once a product and agent of history, a site of experience, memory, storytelling, and aesthetic judgment. The subject is an agent of knowing and of action and the conflicted site for moral acts and gestures. "Modes of subjectivation are determined by the vagaries of the state, family and community hierarchies, medical and scientific experiments and markets. Yet subjectivity is not just the outcome of social control or the unconscious; it also provides the ground for subjects to think through their circumstances and to feel through their contradictions" (Biehl et al. 2007: 7). Indeed, the subject constitutes him- or herself by drawing on complex and contradictory forces involving local cultural practices, interpersonal relationships, and socioeconomic processes in politically and historically specific contexts. In these processes, individuals construct, negotiate, and contest their social experiences and identities.

Psychiatry provides people with concepts through which to conceive of themselves and with techniques for care, healing, and self-fashioning; such concepts and techniques influence the lifelong processes of self-formation (cf. Hacking 1986). With its biomedical baseline, psychiatry conceives of patients as biological and biochemical organisms. When a patient is diagnosed as suffering from a certain mental disorder and prescribed psychopharmaceutical drugs, the medical framework and the medication itself influence his or her subjectivity. Yet patients or their families may deploy alternative treatment models or culturally salient narratives to assert a preferred sense of self, one that is relational and social. This fuller "self" may allow the patient or relatives to create shared meanings with others, or to render the illness experience intelligible. In this process, the selfhood assumed in psychiatry and that found in alternative therapeutic resources or in the local cultural settings interact with and illuminate one another.[1]

Since China's market economy was introduced in the 1980s, Chinese psychiatry has increasingly relied on psychopharmacological treatment (Lee 2011; Ma 2012). Policy changes in 2005 gave Chinese patients access to modern antidepressants and antipsychotics from abroad. Throughout this period, the emphasis has been on expediting "recovery" in order to minimize the price tag for the state, as well as potential dangers, including violence and disruption, popularly associated in China with mental illness. However, psychiatry has not completely supplanted other illness explanations and alternative therapeutic practices in China. Many people with mental illnesses and their families prefer to interpret their experiences in non-biomedical terms and seek relief from Chinese medical doctors or folk healers (Li and Phillips 1990). Many more people, especially in rural areas, cannot afford long-term psychiatric drugs or hospital care. In general, family members are the main caregivers for this large population. Without family support, mental patients may sometimes be placed in welfare facilities (e.g., seniors' homes). Others who completely lack resources may receive no care at all. They must survive on their own, many eventually succumbing to hunger or exposure.

Psychiatrists in China have increasingly adapted to international standards of psychiatric categories and classification, such as the *Diagnostic and Statistical Manual of Mental Disorders* and the *International Classification of Disease*. This openness to new perspectives on mental illness culminated in the release in 2001 of the current third version of the *Chinese Classification of Mental Disorders* (CCMD-3). Sing Lee (2011) points out that the release reflected a break by Chinese mental health leaders from an earlier generation of experts trained mainly in the Russian system of psychiatry. The CCMD-3 system acknowledges the global predominance of Western psychiatry and psychotherapy associated with an increased usage of psychopharmacology. The system also provides a unique opportunity to reflect on the nosological assumptions of Western psychiatry and the changing reality of illness in China.

Take the illness category of schizophrenia, for example. Little research yet describes the cognitive symptoms in Chinese schizophrenic patients, but available studies suggest they are similar to those seen in their Western counterparts (Phillips et al. 1991). This does not, however, mean that culture plays no role in the patterning of symptoms in schizophrenia. One study found that the content of the delusions experienced by schizophrenic patients in China has changed in step with social change (Xia et al. 1990), a finding that resonates with my observations at ZYH. Xia and colleagues also conducted detailed assessment of 448 schizophrenic patients at admission to hospital using a Chinese version of the Scale for Assessment of Positive Symptoms. They found that Chinese patients are more likely than their Western counterparts to experience erotomanic delusions (9.4 percent) and delusions of control (20.8 percent), and are less likely to experience thought broadcasting (7.4 percent), thought withdrawal (5.1 percent), and thought insertion (4.5 percent).

The uniqueness of the practice of psychiatry in China also manifests in rhetoric and methods adopted by Chinese psychiatrists when implementing the biomedical model. At ZYH, Dr. Wen, a chief psychiatrist, used the metaphor of alcohol consumption (a familiar habit in the region) to address concerns by patients and their family members about the side-effects of long-term medication and whether it would leave toxic or harmful residues within a patient's body.

> When alcohol enters the body, it impacts the central nervous system, causing diminished consciousness and unusual behaviors, not unlike psychotic symptoms. But after some time, when the alcohol is metabolized, the symptoms lessen and eventually disappear. The same occurs in the working of drugs, the effects of which will be gradually reduced and won't become long-lasting residues piled up in the body.

Dr. Wen had little difficulty persuading patients to take drugs. Yet he regularly expressed helplessness over the high relapse rate among them. He told me that he had witnessed former patients acting "crazily" in public. Thus, while his metaphors are simple and effective, Dr. Wen could not completely vouch for the efficacy of the drugs that were the backbone of his treatment approach.

Some patients at ZYH, frustrated by their slow recovery, visited bigger hospitals in the provincial capital of Jinan or in Beijing hoping for better treatment. One of them, named Le (ZYH-2012-p19), told me on his return from Jinan that the diagnosis and prescription were almost the same in both Jinan and Zhangqiu, where ZYH is based, except the dose of medication prescribed at the bigger hospitals was smaller, and it took longer to see a specialist psychiatrist and involved more complicated procedures. Since then, Le has been satisfied back at ZYH, but is saddened and frustrated that doctors in all settings concur on the likelihood that he will have to take drugs for life to treat his bipolar disorder.

Indeed, dosing of psychopharmaceutical drugs and their possible side-effects constituted a site of negotiation and contestation among patients, family members, and psychiatrists in the settings where I studied. Let us return to Lili (MKH-2015-p6), the MKH patient whom we discussed in the previous chapter. Now in her early thirties, Lili has experienced symptoms of schizophrenia since her university years. During the first few years of her illness, she saw various specialists in almost all of the Beijing hospitals, but none of those psychiatrists' prescriptions worked for her; she suffered constant relapses – delusion, insomnia, and non-stop talking day and night. Finally, as noted in Chapter 4, one of her father's friends introduced her to a psychiatrist at MKH, Dr. Yuan, who prescribed her the same types of drugs but in a much bigger dose, which finally worked. The side-effects were, of course, much stronger. But Dr. Yuan's rationale is to first control the symptoms and then gradually reduce the dose. He explained, "The side-effects will eventually come under control, but the fear of possible side-effects cannot become the reason to indulge the symptoms, which are more detrimental." Dr. Yuan and many other psychiatrists I spoke to in my research did not aim to construct their patients as *zhengchang ren* (normal people, normalizing patients by eradicating their symptoms), but to return them to society as *shehui ren* (social people: who are socially functioning with mitigated symptoms on medication). Thus, for these psychiatrists, while the primary sense of subjectivity is a well-functioning biochemical being, in practice, they accept and even work on the socially functioning person. Subjectivity is complicated even in biomedical terms, entailing both the biological and the social being.

Lili and her parents seemed satisfied with Dr. Yuan's prescription – at least Lili's symptoms were under control and she could manage a "normal" life independently. However, to offset the side-effects, including weight gain, listlessness, and nausea, Lili's mother had been trying various ways to enhance her daughter's immune system, strengthen her constitution and overall health, as well as enlarge the scope of her subjective sense of her own possibilities. Included in Lili's mother's efforts were Chinese herbal medicine, a nutritious diet, and physical exercise. Following the suggestion of a Chinese medical doctor, Lili had seven raw chestnuts in the morning and seven before dinner to boost her *qi* (life force, often carried through blood: see Chen 2003), which, according to this doctor, was ruined by the psychotic drugs. In addition, this doctor invited Lili to join her to practice Tai Chi and introduced her to a hiking group for more exercise and social interaction.

Lili's mother turned to Chinese medicine as a supplement in part because it adopts a more holistic approach to subjects who experience mental disorders. It conceives of physiology as a dynamic and organic process involving the interactions of energies and forces from both inside and outside the body and the self. As Chinese medicine explains it, madness can proceed as follows: normally the life force or *qi* flows smoothly. When heart-emotion is constrained, the closely related liver *qi* becomes stagnant; stagnant *qi* is then transformed into fire, which dries up bodily fluids and produces phlegm congestion; the fire consumes heart-blood, and the *yin* or fluid aspect of the heart system is depleted; *yin* depletion leads to rampant fire – the usual pattern of *qi* stagnation (*yuzheng*) and source of a type of emotional disorder, which can transform into madness (Zhang 2007).

Lili and her parents were not fully aware of the mental illness diagnostics from Chinese medicine, but they appreciated its efficacy in nurturing life "organically." They also recognized that from a Chinese perspective, the health and well-being of the heart relied on relationships with others. Thus, while Lili may always require drugs for her condition, her subjectivity is redrawn and enlarged through her parents' personal care, as well as the holistic attentions of Chinese medicine. In my interviews, Lili rued her bad luck in developing this condition and the negative drug side-effects. She felt lousy and sleepy, often canceling social events sponsored by her employer and other outings. Lili experienced a reduced self by having to cut social connections and limit her experience. However, it is unlikely that psychiatrists in China will expand their practice to include holistic interventions, even though they clearly care about their patients' wellness, because holistic work is costly and demands more of a doctor's time. Further, there is an alignment between the reduced subjectivity of the medicated person and the subjectivity promoted by the larger turn in China toward therapeutic governance: that subject is more independent and entrepreneurial, endeavoring to find and apply practical measures (in this case, pharmaceuticals) to return to productivity as quickly as possible. The Chinese state, while making legal advances to protect the rights of mentally ill people, delivers them to a mental health care system that tends to facilitate or re-create the conditions of an increasingly neoliberal market.

## PSYCHIATRIC CARE AT TWO MENTAL HOSPITALS

MKH in Beijing, sponsored by China's Ministry of Civil Affairs, is designed to treat the mental health of vulnerable groups. This hospital seems more sensitive and better equipped to protect patient privacy and implement humanitarian treatment than ZYH at Zhangqiu. At MKH, locked iron doors, which create a prison-like atmosphere at ZYH, have been replaced with password-controlled glass doors, giving patients a sense of openness and freedom. The usual iron window bars to prevent patient escape have been transformed at MKH into pleasing ironwork flowers. Video surveillance is not allowed in sleeping quarters to protect patient privacy. With its greater financial resources, MKH avoids the odors that plague ZYH by disposing of anything that cannot be machine-washed, and by hiring more cleaning staff to enforce higher sanitation standards. MKH also has a separate section accommodating seniors with dementia and their privately hired caregivers, compared to ZYH, which has no such capacity; people with dementia there are intermixed with the population of mentally ill people.

Relations between staff and patients in Chinese mental hospitals are not without tensions: there is occasional mistreatment of patients and accidents are not unknown; the secure glass enclosing the worktable of psychiatric nurses, meanwhile, highlights possible dangers from "violent" patients. Nevertheless, nurses at both hospitals interact with and care for patients intimately on a daily basis. At MKH, for example, one game the nurses often organize for patients is *youdian da hongzha* (virtues/merits brainstorming). Each patient is asked to name the virtues of another patient. The patient who is praised then jots down all of the virtues others have identified and reads them aloud. In addition, every day patients are asked to read two recovery stories. Both activities aim to help patients enhance their self-esteem and regain confidence in their recovery. At the same time, they can also be seen as a form of surveillance by nurses, who seek to learn each patient's attitude toward their illness, gain a better understanding of their ideological state, and better assess their recovery progress so they can adjust (typically drug-based) treatments. Nurses told me that morning exercises are considered the most popular activity among patients, with the highest attendance rate (over 90 percent of patients at MKH), and are designed to relax patients and enhance their constitution, but also to temporarily distract them from their symptoms and from any intra-patient and patient–staff tensions. At MKH, several nurses likewise emphasized the value of communication (*goutong*) with patients in helping them to "recover" – that is, become socially functioning with diminished symptoms due to drug regimens, rather than symptom-free – but also in maintaining order on the wards. For example, patients sometimes believe nurses are trying to harm them and refuse medications. Nurses at MKH observed these patients carefully in order to find a breakthrough.

In general, psychiatric nurses and psychiatrists in both hospitals with whom I spoke believed that patients sense kindness and tend to return it. For patients, kindness toward care workers had different motivations, including strategic avoidance of forceful confinement or other modes of control. While both ZYH and MHK mainly rely on psychopharmacology, MKH also has a small psychological counseling division (ZYH offers nearly no talk therapy) staffed by four medical doctors-turned-counselors who sometimes collaborate with the psychiatrists in diagnosing and treating patients. In such combined diagnoses, counselors may identify key psychological issues manifested in patient narratives. However, the counseling sessions are always short (about 20 minutes) and end with psychiatrists prescribing drugs to the clients. One female outpatient I interviewed at MKH indicated that the talk therapy was too short for her to reveal the whole story of how she developed distress. Also, with two doctors present at the same time, the "counseling" session was not sufficiently intimate, and at some point she even felt like she was being interrogated by both physicians. Continuous counseling sessions have been occasionally offered to inpatients at MKH, but for outpatients such sessions become time-consuming and cost-prohibitive. As limited as it is, inpatient counseling does offer a less reductive environment for treatment than that available at ZYH.

At ZYH, my interviews with patients and psychiatric care workers present a complex picture that ties psychiatric treatment to the uneven distribution of mental health care through drugs and the recognized forms of subjectivity that focus on the "healthy" (i.e., socially engaged, productive) rationale, but ultimately detach individuals associated with drug therapy (and therapeutic governance). According to Dr. Wen, ZYH facilities have long been dilapidated and overcrowded. Patients have often been turned away owing to limited capacity. During my visits, the residential wards of ZYH were mostly quiet. But I did witness cases where men were forcefully pulled into the building by family members, and once saw a young girl crying, fighting, and accusing her parents of putting her in the hospital against her will. Another time I saw a nurse involved in a similarly forceful hospitalization. Dr. Wen indicated that he is often called to family homes by the parents of patients to help hospitalize loved ones in extreme distress. He is also called upon by doctors from other general hospitals in Zhangqiu to help treat patients who suffer both physical and mental illness.

At ZYH, the reductive psychopharmacological approach is supplemented by attempts on the part of doctors and patients to enlarge the subjectivities of patients through, for example, personal attention or occasional talk therapy. However, they are ultimately bound to the drug-based system. To some extent, any psychological care there can be viewed as a way to facilitate the smooth operation of psychopharmacological care. In this way, mental health "care" is reminiscent of the "care" that the Chinese state supports within its current mode of therapeutic governance. For example, when community psychosocial workers coach unemployed workers to be positive and self-reliant, their efforts are both genuine and embedded within a framework in which the coaching is intended to relieve the state of responsibility for mass layoffs or sustained welfare support.

One of my informants was a single woman named Wan in her fifties who has suffered from schizophrenia since her thirties (ZYH-2015-p11). She first developed symptoms simultaneously with a failed relationship with a boyfriend and has long believed this man to be her husband, telling people he went to Mars as a firefighter. During her stay at ZYH in March 2015, she would nervously pace the corridor during visiting hours, repeatedly asking nurses why her husband had not come to see her. When nurses told her that her husband had gone to Hainan Province for earthquake relief, or to Iraq to fight for world peace, she seemed satisfied with these explanations and returned to her room. Through such personal care, the nurses tried to make up for failures in biomedicine. At other times, nurses took patients outside for fresh air. They had divided the space behind the residential care building into a makeshift basketball court and a vegetable garden where patients could play and plant vegetables.

On the women's ward, it was so cold and damp during my interviews in November that the head nurse gave me a small hot-water bottle for my hands, which I shared with various patient informants. Several of them made a point of telling me how this gesture touched them, saying that I treated them as human. A number of them revealed that they were sometimes forcefully confined to their beds, even when they were not violent. Others complained that they were forced by nurses to take cold showers (the solar heating system did not work properly in cloudy weather) even when they were menstruating.

At the time of my research, ZYH had only one three-story building, constructed in 1990. The division of patients is based on age and gender, rather than illness category. The ground floor is for senior patients, the second floor for women, and the third floor is for male patients. Over 85 percent of the patients suffer from symptoms of schizophrenia. Each room is designed to hold five beds, but now holds seven. Families generally pay for care. During my observations, I knew of two patients who were sent to the hospital by their township government because they had been traveling to Beijing repeatedly to petition for "imaginary" causes. Beijing police had reassigned them to the local government, which in turn committed them to ZYH.

## BIOMEDICINE OR TALK THERAPY?

At ZYH, Dr. Wen, director and chief psychiatrist, enjoys a good reputation as a caring, attentive, and efficacious doctor. He was trained in internal medicine two decades ago in Shandong Province. Because of his keen interest in mental health, he then shifted his focus to psychiatry. Now he has the largest number of patients at ZYH, seeing between 30 and 50 people daily, including both new and returning patients. He holds consultations with and diagnoses patients one by one on a "first come, first served" basis in the presence of other patients and family members. In his office setting, there is no way of achieving privacy for patients. Dr. Wen is fully aware of this problem, which he highlighted in an application for funds to expand ZYH. Each consultation begins by Dr. Wen asking the patient and his or her accompanying friend or family members a few questions, soliciting key symptoms. Based on these symptoms, he writes a diagnosis in the patient-record booklet (*menzhen guiding*) without asking why the patient has had a particular feeling, or whether he or she has recently experienced any traumatic life events. Often within less than 10 minutes the patient receives a diagnosis and prescription, and Dr. Wen directs them to the hospital pharmacy.

Dr. Wen's main task is to explain to the patient how to take the prescribed medicine: which pill is taken at what time, and when to reduce the quantity of the medication – taking half a pill when the patient experiences certain symptoms, then further reducing the dose to one quarter of the pill if the patient experiences another set of symptoms. He writes down these directions on the labels of the drugs bottles. While diagnosing patients in his office, Dr. Wen also takes phone calls via both his cell phone and his office phone, making appointments, giving directions to other patients who are not present on how to take medicine, or explaining whether certain side-effects are normal. As director of ZYH, he explained, his cell phone is to be on at all times.

While Dr. Wen claimed that he could do psychological counseling, during my participant observation his counseling remained minimal in order to complete diagnosis and see everyone waiting for him that day. One morning in November 2015, as I was observing in Dr. Wen's office, a woman in her late forties wept on a corner of the couch while repeatedly stifling a cough. When it was her turn, her husband did most of the talking, explaining that his wife had not been able to sleep for five days and nights, crying all the time. When Dr. Wen asked how she felt, the woman, while weeping, started to talk: "I have a heavy headache, nausea, and feel dizzy all the time." Her husband interrupted: "She loses her temper easily and is very confrontational these days. You say one sentence and she responds with 10." His weeping wife snapped at him, "It's a big family, so much housework; no one cares about how I feel …" Again interrupting his wife and probably trying to prevent her revealing too much of their family matters in public, her husband jumped in, saying, "See, doctor, see, she didn't have the patience to listen to me." His wife did not challenge him, but continued weeping. Even while listening to their conversation, Dr. Wen was writing down his diagnosis. He said with a level tone, "Well, I think you as a husband perhaps come on too strong; you should at least let your wife finish her talk." Then, immediately showing the couple his diagnosis, which he had written into the woman's patient-record booklet, he said to the husband, rather than to the wife, in a way that infantilized the latter, "OK, I give you a small dose of medication to help her sleep; she needs sleep, otherwise she cannot function normally, and something to stabilize her mood." He then pointed them to the hospital pharmacy.

While Dr. Wen is fully aware of the limitations of the clinical setting for talk therapy and for protecting patients' privacy, he insists that he tries to make his diagnoses as precise and efficacious as possible. After all, the doctor's basic responsibility, as he claimed, is to alleviate the suffering of patients and to provide immediate relief. Here, biomedical reductionism takes on a moral dimension: each patient only has about five minutes to present his or her symptoms; Dr. Wen considers it his duty to do his best within these constraints. These limitations effectively occluded the deeper causes of distress, which, arguably, the Chinese government and its agents are ethically obliged to address. Indeed, suffering is the very link between patients and doctors. In this way, Dr. Wen's practice highlights the narrow focus of therapeutic governance, which exerts control through narrow forms of care, targeted at the individual, while eliding other forms of care – including structural change and wider social support and recognition – that might reduce distress on a large scale.

Yet it seemed easier in the rural setting of ZYH for family members and people with mental illness to see their suffering as relational and social. Schizophrenia again provides a good example. Michael Phillips and colleagues (2000) report that very few patients with schizophrenia in China or their family members consider biological factors important causes. In a study in Suzhou, Jiangsu Province, and Siping, Jilin Province, 245 family members of 135 schizophrenic patients attributed 84 percent of the cause of schizophrenia to social, interpersonal, and psychological problems; no respondent considered schizophrenia a "disease of the brain" (Phillips et al. 2000). They also found that family members of well-educated urban patients are more likely to employ internal attributions, blaming the condition on defects in the patient, such as "personality problems." Family members from rural areas are more likely to use external attributions, blaming the condition on factors outside the patient's control, such as spiritual or mystical forces. While I did not encounter patients or family members who blamed spiritual or mystical forces for symptoms, I did often hear patients attribute their conditions to social and interpersonal factors. One afternoon in April 2015, just before Dr. Wen closed his office, I was able to talk with his last patient of that day, a woman in her late forties named Jia who was waiting for her husband to fill her prescription at the on-site pharmacy (ZYH-2015-p15), after which Dr. Wen would explain how to take the drugs. This woman had symptoms associated with schizophrenia. I asked how and when she developed these symptoms. She stated that her husband had been promoted to division director at the village factory and had become busy socializing at dinners and banquets, returning home late. As a fulltime housewife, she was lonely. Jia started to suspect that her husband was having an affair and stalked him at his factory, trying to find out who his mistress was. After her failure to identify a mistress, she started to hallucinate and hear voices of a man who looked like one of her male classmates from junior high school. Later, her husband confirmed that after her failure to catch his mistress, whose existence he denied, she became temperamental and confrontational at home, obsessing over talks with her "boyfriend" day and night. In this case, the change of her husband's status, loneliness, and fear for the loss of her relationship contributed to her mental distress. For Jia, talking to her "classmate" was neither good or bad, but rather a strategy to cope with emptiness and loneliness. In her mind, being forced to take drugs not only demonstrated her husband's jealousy and narrow-mindedness, but also caused her constant nausea and listlessness. She indicated that if her husband were to stop seeing his mistress and stay home more, she would stop interacting with her "classmate." In this sense, Jia viewed her delusionary talk as revenge, and her distress as largely based on an estranged relationship with her husband, rather than as a sickness that could be fixed with drugs.

## TALK THERAPY AS RESISTANCE AGAINST PSYCHOPHARMACOLOGY

When I first visited the iron-barred women's ward at ZYH in the summer of 2012, Dr. Wen introduced me as a researcher interested in mental health seeking input from patients regarding their experiences and insights. Quite a few were excited at the opportunity to talk and, in fact, none thought that they were really ill. One patient, a woman in her late thirties named Xia (ZYH-2012-p5; also see below) told me,

> This [talk therapy] is what I had thought the hospital would offer but after I came here, no one has ever talked with me about my experiences, even asking me how I was coping. What they do is make sure that we take the medicine on time; we have to open our mouths to assure them that we did swallow our pills without hiding them under our tongues. Now I've become a "medicine pot" [yao guanzi]. The medicine makes me feel numb and dizzy … I was sharp before.

Xia explicitly challenged the predominant psychopharmacological approach to hospital care, which centered her life on a drug treatment schedule, rendering her subjectivity mainly as biomedical.

One day in November 2015, while I was sitting in Dr. Wen's office taking notes on his consultations and diagnoses, a woman in her late thirties named Chen (ZYH-2015-p10) suddenly moved to sit next to me, asking if she could speak with me informally. She obviously mistook me for the director's assistant. I asked why she would not wait to talk with the doctor. She whispered to me, "Too many people. It's not good for talk. Obviously he only prescribes pills, does not talk. I want to talk, having too much buried in my chest. Taking drugs will get you addicted, more symptoms." I then told the woman I was not the doctor's assistant and could not diagnose, but I was happy to talk with her. After we exchanged phone numbers, she left.

I met Chen again on a Sunday afternoon. She briefly told me that she suffered from symptoms of depression, with almost the same symptoms as her ex-boyfriend, who used to be treated by Dr. Wen. She said she did not want to get as addicted to psychopharmaceutical drugs as her ex-boyfriend, and preferred counseling. This perception – that people can be addicted to psychopharmaceuticals – was common among family and patients, and correlated with the lack of talk therapy. Some evidence from China shows that counseling can work better than drugs, at least in the treatment of depression. A recent study reveals that the recovery rate of depression through psychopharmaceutical drugs is between 22 and 40 percent, but as high as 42 to 66 percent if treatment focuses on or includes cognitive behavioral therapy.[2] However, medication is more accessible and cheaper than counseling, especially for China's rural population.

In addition to contesting biomedicine through a preference for talk therapy or psychological care, patients challenged reductive psychiatry through a range of other genres, for example the agency demonstrated in their delusional narratives. Xia (ZYH-2012-p5) spoke quickly and rationally. If not for meeting her at a mental hospital, I would never have guessed that she had suffered from schizophrenia for over five years. Her symptoms included hallucination and hearing voices. Her admission to ZYH in November 2015 was because she had heard a voice that she thought was Dr. Wen, her psychiatrist for years, appointing her to work at ZYH by saying, "Ayaya, you finally came. We find you an excellent doctor!" After hearing this voice several times, Xia came to ZYH, telling Dr. Wen that she accepted his offer. Dr. Wen was both surprised and amused. He called Xia's father, who said Xia had forced her mother to give her money to study psychiatry at Qingdao Medical School because she wanted to become a psychiatrist.

When Xia talked with me at ZYH's women's ward, she said that having been so frequently admitted to ZYH, and having interacted with other patients and psychiatrists, she knew how to diagnose people with mental illness. "When the prescribed drugs do not work on your symptoms, they give you different ones. We basically become a testing ground for their experimental treatment." In my three in-depth interviews with her, Xia could pinpoint key defining symptoms of schizophrenia, depression, bipolar disorders, body dysmorphic disorder, and other mental disorders. She could precisely associate these symptoms with her inpatient friends at ZYH. While she acknowledged that she did not know about drug dosing or specific drug function, this part of psychopharmaceutical knowledge could be easily acquired, considering that the doctors at ZYH sometimes experimented by giving patients different prescriptions and different doses until something worked. This flexibility of her doctors' treatments made Xia think she too could master psychiatry. She was perplexed by her doctors' doubts in this regard. She looked and sounded certain, confident, and clear-minded. Given her educational background as a junior high school graduate, this confidence may seem misplaced. Still, Xia's aspiration offers a critique of the reductionism and experimentalism of psychiatric treatment at ZYH, which she has experienced first-hand.

## SIDE-EFFECTS AS SITES OF NEGOTIATION AND CONTESTATION

Unlike patients in Guangdong Province, who have been shown to deploy Chinese medicine and religion as major forms of cultural resistance against Western psychiatry (Ma 2012), my informants in both Beijing and Shandong never completely rejected biomedicine, despite complaining about the side-effects of psychopharmaceutical drugs. Instead, they actively looked for ways to minimize or offset side-effects. In fact, none of my informants relied exclusively on Chinese medicine or other alternative healing resources (cf. Ma 2012) to treat severe psychiatric diseases such as bipolar disorder, major depressive disorder, or schizophrenia. Instead they used Chinese medicine or other alternative healing resources in conjunction with psychopharmacology in order to cope with drug side-effects. In this way, for them, the potential and actual side-effects of biomedicine constitute a site of negotiation and contestation.

Returning to the example of schizophrenia, we can see that it also offers a window onto this contestation. In China, as in many developing countries, the primary responsibility for caring and managing a schizophrenic illness falls to the family (not the state or the health system). Traditionally, family members in China assume responsibility for all the health care decisions of a seriously ill individual (see Chiang 2014); in the case of schizophrenia, the decisions that must be made are complex and require significant assessment of biomedical and alternative possibilities for care. Families are thus engaged, from the beginning, in cobbling together forms of care that work, preserving as much of the full subjectivity of their loved ones as possible, and dealing with changes in their relationships with them once they undergo drug therapy. Indeed, among family members of 456 Chinese schizophrenic patients, 65 percent reported that the illness had a severe effect on healthy family members' emotional well-being over the prior three months, while 46 percent reported a severe effect on healthy family members' work (Phillips et al. 1998).

To return to an example from Chapter 4, the case of Sun (ZYH-2015-p6) and her husband, Zhang Jilin, 62, who has suffered from schizophrenia for over 35 years, captures these difficulties. Sun emphasized to me that her husband's schizophrenia was a job injury. Thirty-five years ago, a collapse at the coal mine where he worked buried a co-worker. Zhang, together with his co-workers, dug for over 24 hours to recover his friend's corpse. Zhang soon suffered symptoms of acute stress disorder and then schizophrenia. Sun insisted that she had single-handedly cared for her husband for over three decades without payment or social recognition. She did not hesitate to send her husband to hospital in cases of emergency, but she did not easily trust hospital care after traumatic experiences there. About eight years ago, when her husband suffered a major relapse, she had to send him to LWH, a mental hospital in Shandong Province designated by Zhang's former employer, the coal-mining company. Sun showed me a photo of her husband from that period. In it, Zhang stood against the wall at the ward, gaunt, bald, and dirty. In his fifties at the time, he looked thirty years older. Yet Sun said he had been vibrant, with thick hair, when he had first been admitted, just two months before. When Sun visited him, his legs were severely swollen, as were his feet, which were glued to his shoes by the fluid that oozed from them. He was downcast and he smelled, crying for Sun to take him home. He said that the big black pills he had to take every other day would kill him; the medication was so strong that it would make him sleep for two days. Sun said,

> I was so outraged that I ran to the doctors' office yelling at the two doctors there, "Why has my husband become this way?" "What did you do to make a big man shrink so much?" "What did he do to deserve being tortured this way?" He came here only mentally ill; now he is ill both physically and mentally! I collected his stuff and immediately took him out of the hospital. … This is hell for a human! I kept this picture and may sue them.

After so many years of caring for her husband, Sun has concluded that medication alone does not work; her husband needs "psychological care." Sun believes in the value of counseling and family care in relieving Zhang's symptoms. She insists that her own care is why Zhang is the only survivor of the original 36 mental patients sent to LWH through his former employer.

According to Sun, it took over half a year to partially neutralize the side-effects of Zhang's stay there. The drugs and their side-effects, which had destroyed Zhang's health and vitality, have become Sun and Zhang's explicit and implicit "enemy," one they fight together on a daily basis. Whenever Zhang refuses to eat certain nutritional supplements or take a walk for his overall health, Sun employs a rhetoric of helping him fight or cope with the heavy blow of the medication. Like Lili's mother, Sun sometimes boiled Chinese herbal medicine to help Zhang boost his immunity, not as an alternative to his medication for schizophrenia but as a supplement. For Zhang, the side-effects of psychiatric medication have also become a motivation to work with more traditional resources to achieve a relatively healthy lifestyle. Sun is proud of her perseverance and moral integrity in staying in her marriage and caring for her husband for over three decades. She has reflected that, if she had suffered schizophrenia, she doubts that her husband would have stayed to care for her for so long.

As Arthur Kleinman (2009) points out, caregiving is a moral practice. It is "a practice of empathic imagination, responsibility, witnessing and solidarity with those in great need." Kleinman also sees caregiving as a humanizing practice, as "one of those relationships and practices of self-cultivation that make us, even as we experience our limits and failures, more human. It completes … our humanity" (2009: 293).

Negotiation includes whether one takes drugs at all, what the dosage is, or whether one stays in a hospital or not. Since the drugs are helpful to some degree, the use of other resources offers a way to mitigate side-effects and retain the direct benefits of the medication.

## INTIMATE AND AUTHORITATIVE PSYCHIATRIC CARE

One of the unique developments I observed in both research settings of Beijing and Shandong Province is the intimate relationship between psychiatrists and patients that preserves physician authority while going beyond a normative, professional doctor–patient boundary. Such relationships may be partly derived from the Chinese cultural context, in which kinship is the basis of social organization and social imagination. Therapeutic relationships enable psychiatrists to access the private and inner lives – the subjectivities – of their clients more profoundly.

Alternatively, doctors and patients may be working to negotiate better mental health care in the context of the growing mental health indus-try, where psychopharmaceutical drugs are a quick fix.

At ZYH, Dr. Wen has developed a kind of paternal clientelism with some of his former patients. One of these, Ming (ZYH-2015-p16), a teenager, has suffered from schizophrenia for about three years. During every visit, Ming and his father would first wait outside Dr. Wen's office until other patients had gone, and then come in to spend some quality time with the doctor, whom Ming calls "uncle." Ming would show Dr. Wen his new gadgets and the new computer games he played, mean-while describing recent developments in his life. Ming's father calls Dr. Wen whenever the boy refuses to take medication or in situations that both parents are unable to handle. With a brief talk with his "uncle" and doctor, this boy is soon at ease and peaceful, and does whatever he is asked. In general, Dr. Wen is kind and attentive to patients. The only time in three summers that I saw him raise his voice was when a middle-aged woman refused to take medication for fear of possible side-effects and argued with him in front of a dozen patients. Dr. Wen scolded the woman, telling her firmly, "I would rather you eat delicious meat and fish all the time but that could not cure your symptoms. If you don't want to take medication, then you don't need to come to see me again; I don't know how to treat you." With these words, he further stressed his psychopharmacological approach. The rare outburst, however, delineated the limits of Dr. Wen's practice, which, arguably, parallel those of therapeutic governance in general. At its heart, the deployment of medicalized care as a tool of governance is a means to pragmatically exert control without undertaking the costly process of addressing deeper issues – such as the "side-effects" of socioeconomic change.

Still, Dr. Wen took pride in befriending many of his (former) patients and helping them solve both mental and pragmatic issues. One of these, a man named Huang, whom he had treated for bipolar disorder, called him one day from another city. While visiting that city, Huang got into a fight with another tourist. During the confrontation, he produced a fruit knife to scare the man, who consequently called the police. Huang was then taken to the local police station. During the interrogation, Huang recalled his history of mental illness, informing the police of his condition. The police then called Dr. Wen to confirm his story and subsequently released Huang without charge. With this example, Dr. Wen tried to emphasize that in addition to medical assistance, he offers pragmatic help. Indeed, despite his focus on reductive psychopharmacology, he enjoys a sense that his (former) patients have well-rounded subjectivities grounded in the real social world, and he occasionally makes efforts to enrich these subjectivities through personal care.

## CONCLUSION

Through this ethnographic account of the uneven development and distribution of psychiatric care services in two Chinese hospitals, I have examined the interactions between psychopharmaceutical drugs and individual subjectivities in China, and how individuals experience psychotropic drugs at the intersection of biological, sociocultural, and structural forces by considering their illness experiences as involving agency, morality, and social relationships (see Kleinman 1995; Jenkins 2011). I have also demonstrated that psychiatry in contemporary China is situated at a contentious intersection of several key forces, including the cultural meanings of mental illness, institutional practices, and national interests – such as the interest within therapeutic governance in highlighting narrow definitions of "care." The analysis also takes account of the complex subject formation occurring in relation to therapeutic and institutional power among the mentally ill. The personalized forms of care that attempt to enrich the subjectivities of people in mental distress emerge from both families and practitioners, who, paradoxically, work within psychiatric institutions. Families attempt to maintain a richer subjective experience for those on drugs, and even doctors and nurses do their best to enlarge subjectivity through personal attention, but they are restrained by a system that narrowly focuses on treating distress with medication. Even psychiatric labels can negatively impact people's lives. For example, the discourse around major depression puts patients in situations where they are simultaneously told that they can conquer depression if they continue treatment and that depression is a lifelong affliction inherent in their neurochemical makeup. The only way of escaping a life course of continued treatment and self-management is to reject both the disease category and the treatment, a situation that might be liberating for patients or dangerous if it ends up isolating them yet further. I suggest that this situation should compel debate on a reorientation of psychiatry in China toward reform or through anti-psychiatric critique.

Psychiatry in China shares an aim with the state for modernization, rationalization, and global integration. Downplaying social contributions to mental distress simultaneously results from and legitimizes the lack of state social support and the unbalanced treatment model that relies solely on drugs. A more balanced model would include counseling, drugs, and a progressive, social-justice approach to care for mentally distressed people, especially those on the margins of Chinese society. By emphasizing mind–body dualism, psychiatry seeks to produce an ideally modern self that is bounded in the healthy self, guided by the rational mind, and detached from social or cultural ties. This contrasts with the expanded versions of subjectivity that include social identities, social others, bodily needs like exercise, and more. Deemed an efficacious force liberating individuals mired in their social and economic worlds, psychiatry transforms them into modern selves who can switch their minds on and off via biochemical regulation. In short, biomedical somatization decouples individuals from their social and cultural reality and reduces them to biomedical or biochemical beings. Nikolas Rose (2006) suggests that psychiatry has promoted a self-understanding informed by neurochemical knowledge and genetic susceptibility to particular diseases. This neurochemical self in the Chinese context is enforced through state-sponsored insurance, institutional control, and "socialization." Instead of normalizing patients by helping them eradicate their symptoms, psychiatrists insist that they try to make them social persons again: that is, help them to return to their social functions while possibly still keeping their (mitigated) symptoms.

Patients and their families contest, defy, and resist this bare subjectivity, employing alternative or complementary therapeutic resources, as well as agentive uses of life techniques, ethical standards, or folk wisdom based on Chinese traditions or embedded in the culture of a community. These complicated processes defy the unified, socially detached individual who is often the recipient of biomedical treatment and perceptions of an exclusively somatic self constructed by psychiatry. Indeed, the biomedical perspective in China does include a social dimension, as patients are judged to be healing if they can function in society despite their symptoms and medication (in the case of Lili). In the next chapter, I will continue to chart this social dimension through analysis of the ways Chinese cultural traditions such as Buddhism, Confucianism, and Daoism integrate as healing resources into psychotherapeutic practices.

# 6 | Counseling and Indigenous Psychology

Without medication, talk can relieve patients' symptoms.
*A physician-turned-counselor in Beijing*

When you encounter difficulties in life, the solutions are often hidden in
your heart; it is a counselor's task to help you dig them out.
*A counselor in Beijing*

Over the past two decades, psychological counseling has surged in
China. The field includes a range of traditions, methods, and techniques. As elsewhere, counseling is practiced in China with varying
degrees of professionalism in multiple settings; it is a hybrid, mixing
indigenous and Western forms of psychotherapeutic theories and techniques. However, Chinese counseling in its many forms has developed
in synergy with local society and its practice has characteristically
Chinese personal and political implications. In this chapter, I consider both. I analyze several indigenous counseling methods currently in practice: *shudao liaofa* (dredging therapy), *yixiang duihua
liaofa* (imagery communication psychotherapy, or ICP), *juying* ("giant
infant") therapy, a unique mixed method of anger management, and
folk or faith healing. I show how these methods, which simultaneously draw on and critique Western psychotherapy, do paradoxical
work: while counseling seeks to enhance people's access to their inner
worlds – people's heart-minds – it also opens those inner worlds to
scrutiny, regulation, or control by experts and the state in the process

of psychoboom and psychologization. However, such control is hegemonic as psychotherapy or therapy in general accesses the subjectivity
of the client through care, compassion, and permissive empathy. In its
various forms, counseling reflects Chinese culture and history, and it
also appears to orient the population for a future in which the party
state authorizes subject formation and identity.

The focus in counseling on cultivating (new) spaces of interiority
for individual growth and autonomy marginalizes the traditional role
of the family and interpersonal harmony in subject formations. That
is, such counseling is oriented toward constructing a self free to engage
in internal mental activity but relatively indifferent to the social world.
In this way, counseling practiced in China resonates with Western
cognitive therapy strategies that privilege the internal, subjective experience of clients, who are encouraged to change their subjective experience of reality rather than work to change their social reality (cf.
Sampson 1981). These practices attempt to construct subjects who are
interested in cultivating the depth of their hearts, unearthing the subconscious realm and potentials, or other aspects of their inner beings
to realize their true selves rather than engaging with broader social,
political, and economic processes.

BACKGROUND: SELF-INTEREST,
OR STATE INTEREST?

Post-1989, the Chinese state sought to re-establish its legitimacy
and stabilize the country. One means to these ends was to endorse a
renewed focus on cultural tradition. For example, a state-sponsored
"Confucianism Craze" (Zhang and Schwartz 1997) arose, through
which people sought comfort and guidance, while simultaneously
renewing a political order based on family, hierarchy, and patriarchy.
For the government, Confucianism is tested for its possible efficacy in
solving contemporary problems and offering alternative technologies for

governing an unevenly developed and increasingly privatized country. State-supported *guoxue dashi* (masters of national studies) have simplified, popularized, and psychologized Confucianism in order to reach a broader audience (Yu 2006; Y. Zhang 2014). By invoking Confucian precepts and doctrines, as well as those of Daoism and Buddhism, the process of "re-traditionalization" moralizes people's psychological readjustment and facilitates certain psychological mechanisms.

Concurrent with this "re-traditionalization," Western psychology is infiltrating the Chinese context like never before, contributing to a market economy that has promoted the psychoboom of psychotherapy, self-help culture, and greater access to psychopharmaceutical drugs (Kleinman 2010). As the middle class expands and competition increases for economic advancement, *peixun* (training) has also been booming. With the goal of providing people with practical skills to get ahead in the job market, *peixun* focuses in great part on improving people's psychological quality and maximizing their potential, particularly through *xintai peixun* (heart-attitude training). In this way, the middle class has been exposed to a new blend of psychology, Confucianism/Buddhism/Daoism, and market strategy.[1]

In parallel with "re-traditionalization" and the psychoboom, the Chinese system of social support underwent major retrenchment. Public funding for health care decreased during the 1990s and beyond, and much of the responsibility for this care was delegated by the central government to local authorities and hospitals, which are more profit-oriented, making mental health services more expensive and less accessible to most Chinese. For example, the first three forms of therapeutic practice I describe below are typically available to those in the middle or upper classes. For people in lower socioeconomic classes, including laid-off workers and rural migrants, resident committees and Party members, who have been trained by the government in psychology and self-help precepts, become purveyors of psychological counseling. Their work, often centering on anger management, stands in for other,

now-defunct forms of social welfare, including stable state employment and health benefits. Thus, the heart-minds of China's working
classes and of the middle class are differently addressed.

## INDIGENOUS PSYCHOLOGY IN CHINA

Louise Sundararajan (2016) defines indigenous psychology (hereafter
IP) as "an intellectual movement across the globe to resist the hegemony of Western psychology in representations of the human mind,
and in investigations of local mentality." IP has many tributaries,
including critical psychology, postcolonial psychology, and psychology
of First Nations. IP consists of two major components: adapting theory
and method from the West and drawing on traditional resources from
the local culture (literature, history, philosophy) for hypothesis testing
and theory construction (Sundararajan 2016). Psychotherapy practiced in China encompasses both. Many Chinese psychologists seek
parallels between Western counseling and Chinese cultural traditions,
including Confucianism, Buddhism, and Daoism, as well as precepts
of "The Art of War." Some counselors I interviewed in Beijing suggested that Confucianism is comparable to humanistic-existential
therapy, given the belief that humans are essentially good (according
to Mencius) and should engage in self-cultivation. Western therapy is
also inflected by "Eastern" practices that emphasize holism and the
body, such as the use of Tibetan singing bowls as a resource for healing
through sound therapy. In general, elements of Chinese cultural traditions are grafted onto Western psychotherapeutic theories and methods
more often than the other way around.

   Chinese counselors I interviewed believe that cultural differences
play a role in designing effective therapy. As illustrated in Chapter 1,
selfhood in China is conceived differently than in the West, recognizing
interdependence in social networks to a greater extent. Whereas
Western psychotherapy addresses feelings in a bounded, masterful,

individualistic self that arises from intrapsychic processes, many Chinese counselors pay greater attention to the body–heart nexus, leading to a sense of a relational or ensemble self. The body is treated as a battlefield of both illnesses and therapy. It is both a healing resource and an entity to be healed. It is also considered as a place to hear the voice of one's heart and to meet one's self. That is, the body acts both as the bridge reaching hearts and as a force transducing other social forces. Well-known Chinese counselor Wu Zhihong, for instance, views counseling as a process to engage *shen xin ling* (the body, heart, and soul). He pays particular attention to the body as a truthful and concrete manifestation of psychological and physical suffering. In one WeChat training session, he remarked:

> Whenever I feel pain, I lie down, feeling my body. … If a certain body part feels the pain stronger, I will dwell on that part for a while. If attention is focused on that part, transformation will occur. That body part will become warm. …While it may be difficult to grasp psychological or spiritual experiences, it is easier to understand our pain and suffering if we feel it directly through the body. (Wu Zhihong 2016)

Wu contends that our mind may cheat us but our body does not lie. It accurately stores all our emotions and wants and reminds us to face our own needs. Indeed, almost all diseases are triggered by negative emotions, and different body parts store or express different emotions. According to Chinese medicine, the kidney is in charge of fear; the liver stores anger, and lungs determine sadness (Hao 2014). Stomach problems may result from pressure or distress; coughing is often caused by fear or anxiety. Physical illnesses are reminders or alarms from the heart – manifestations of deepest longings. Through studying the body and its nuanced changes, one can enjoy a healthier and happier life. Further, sensing distress within the body may actually cause people to behave more ethically. Jun Gu, Chen-Bo Zhong, and

Elizabeth Page-Gould (2013) conducted a series of laboratory studies that suggest people respond to a perception of elevated heartbeat by acting in more principled ways. In other words, the participants tended to interpret somatic symptoms as signals of moral distress and modified their decisions to resolve the moral dilemma. In this regard, experiencing physical symptoms of distress might lead to heightened awareness of the moral dilemmas linked to that distress. The body-focus and more holistic approach in Chinese counseling exemplify the insight within IP that culture inflects psychological practice. However, what is sometimes understudied in IP is the extent to which the dialogic interaction between history and political context also matters. Chinese counseling provides many examples of these inflections. For instance, owing to China's history and post-socialist context, people are accustomed to looking to the authority of the state for direction and guidance, particularly since Mao's era. This history is vital to understanding an element of psychological practice in China today, namely clients' expectation of authoritative, "straightforward" answers to psychological issues, and therapists' readiness to provide instant solutions and pragmatic instructions on how to solve problems and get over stress (Qian et al. 2002). This is why, along with the influence of *peixun* (J. Yang 2015), in recent years counseling in China resembles coaching or training more than typical Western psychotherapy (see Zheng 2009).

Probably for this reason, many psychiatrists or doctors are suspicious of the value of talk therapy altogether. In my interviews in both Beijing and Zhangqiu, psychiatrists saw talk therapy as time-consuming. Likewise, their patients may view "talking" as inefficacious and useless. Dr. Wen from ZYH offered a case to highlight this point. One of his patients, a woman in her late sixties, suffered from insomnia. She suspected her eyeballs were missing and spent nights and nights looking for them in her house. Dr. Wen tried to reconstruct her cognition: if she could see and recognize him at his clinic, she must have eyeballs.

He tried psychoanalysis to seek the subconscious roots of her delusion. But neither logic nor talk therapy satisfied the woman and her husband. Dr. Wen then took a more pragmatic route. He prescribed medication for insomnia and delusion. He also proposed that the woman grow two pots of mint at her door to "protect" her eyeballs (the plant, according to Dr. Wen, releases an appeasing smell). The solution was direct and pragmatic; the lady was happy with the doctor's prescription (taking the medication and growing mint), her symptoms were alleviated, and whatever the source of the problem, it could be conveniently ignored.

History is also vital for understanding other, related aspects of contemporary counseling in China. One key historical concept is that of "thought work": the traditional Communist ideological orientation. Thought work, developed roughly since the 1930s and practiced widely until the mid-1990s, was an ideological ritual through which Party authorities transmitted (and imposed) policies and official ideologies to the rank and file (Rofel 1999; Brady 2008). Many find parallels in thought work with cognitive behavioral therapy (CBT), which is task-based and solution-focused, pragmatic and directive, stressing psychoeducation and homework (Lin 2002; Zhang et al. 2002). It is one of the most popular Western psychotherapeutic methods adopted by Chinese counselors to treat Chinese clients (with anxiety, depression, obsessive compulsive disorder, and post-traumatic stress disorder) because of its adaptability to Chinese culture and specific historical and political contexts (Lin 2002; Guo and Hanley 2015). CBT was developed in the West during the 1960s by incorporating cognitive principles with existing behavioral approaches (Lin 2002; Wills 2010). Its basic assumption is that the ways people think influence the ways they act and feel (Wills 2010). Through CBT, the counselor works with the client to identify, evaluate, and modify maladaptive or "irrational" cognition and behaviors in order to help establish more balanced patterns to regulate the client's thoughts, feelings, and actions.

For example, Derson Young and Yalin Zhang modified a derivation of CBT – rational emotive behavioral therapy – by incorporating Daoist mental health principles and developed Chinese Taoist cognitive psychotherapy (CTCP) in 1992 (Zhang et al. 2002).[2] Daoism is also an influence in the therapies to be discussed below.

Like CBT, thought work aims to reconstruct clients' cognition and consciousness in ways that benefit their "correct" and "rational" thinking and behaviors. Of course, current counseling differs from thought work in other ways: while thought work identified individual interests with collective interests, current counseling asks the individual to draw upon resources of the self, rather than those of the group or the state. Still, the historical resonance with state efforts to transform the self inflects current counseling practice. The emphasis on producing positive-thinking and "rational" subjects still benefits the state in the market economy.

## REVITALIZING CHINESE CULTURAL TRADITIONS AS HEALING RESOURCES

Culture, history, and political realities combine in today's counseling practices in China. The various "indigenous" Chinese therapies approach the inner world of the individuals in ways that are apparently culturally sensitive and familiar. Within Chinese culture, Confucianism and Daoism are two accessible value systems that offer complementary worldviews and modes of coping with the stresses of everyday life. Confucian principles emphasize humanism, social order, filial piety, and moral action, while Daoism emphasizes acceptance, "non-action," or "going with the flow." These value systems shape indigenous Chinese therapies as they continue to take shape today. In general, Buddhism and Daoism have been better integrated into psychotherapy than Confucianism. This may be attributed to China's revitalization of Confucianism as an appendage to its governance. The deployment of

Confucianism de-medicalizes and popularizes psychotherapy, making it part of an everyday ethical practice; it simultaneously moralizes and politicizes counseling owing to the influence of the Chinese state.

*Psychological dredging therapy*

Professor Lu Longguang at the Nanjing Brain Hospital created psychological dredging therapy in 1984.[3] As the first Chinese psychotherapy, *shudao liaofa* (hereafter *shudao*) won multiple awards from the Chinese Ministry of Sciences and of Health. Drawing on precepts on the treatment of mental distress in the "Yellow Emperor's Canon of Internal Medicine" written two thousand years ago as well as precepts of Western psychotherapy, not only does *shudao* claim to suit all kinds of mental disorders, including neuroses, psychosomatic diseases, and psychological disorders, but it can also apply to the general population to improve their psychological well-being. In this therapy, Lu compares possible causes and development of mental disorder to a tree with roots, trunk, and crown (branches and leaves) (see a different tree theory by Xu Kaiwen in Chapter 1). The tree crown represents various symptoms: the trunk represents fear. The roots refer to personality flaws, and the soil in which the tree grows symbolizes individuals' social environment. Because of exposure to certain negative social and cultural contexts, one may develop a flawed personality, encountering difficulties, frustration, and stress. When these challenges cannot be easily overcome, one can develop fears or phobias (*pa*) and symptoms of psychological disorders. Among the two thousand cases he treated, Lu found that the main causes of mental illnesses are personality defects formed as early as infancy (Lu 2006). Self-awareness is the prerequisite for treating psychological disorders. Lu insists that "heartache" (mental distress) needs "heart medicine" such as psychological dredging therapy. Without psychotherapy, mere psychopharmaceutical drugs cannot cure mental disorders.

*Shudao* consists of two processes: one is *shu*, "dredging"; the other is *dao*, "guiding." "Dredging" refers to the effective communications between doctors and patients in order to get rid of any obstacle within the heart-minds of patients for the purpose of promoting their physical and mental health. Through open information exchange, patients are able to expose their psychological problems and cooperate with doctors, going through a psychological conversion process in which their mood changes from negative to positive and their attitude shifts from escaping to facing reality.

*Shudao* entails a three-step dredging process, all of which comes from the precepts of the "Yellow Emperor's Canon of Internal Medicine": first, communication: creating an amicable environment to compel clients to offer autobiographical accounts in order to fully understand possible causes of their mental distress and help them with self-cognition and self-analysis to redress "pathological" attitudes or "twisted" psychology; second, correction: through aversion therapy or other techniques to destroy "ill" mentality or attitudes, counselors then continue to dredge negative feelings or attitudes until the clients themselves can control their "pathological" intentions; and finally, third, guidance: constructing "normal" psychological and behavioral conditions to strengthen healthy psychological dynamics (Lu 2006). The therapeutic model through dredging symptoms is a cycle that gradually deepens clients' cognitive transformation (ignorance → knowing → cognition → practice → effect → re-cognition → re-practice → consolidating therapeutic effects).

*Shudao* shares similar procedures with CBT, paying particular attention to cognitive reconstruction, for instance through face-to-face communication with a doctor or by written letters. The doctors correct some of the "pathological" thoughts or attitudes conveyed in the clients' speeches or letters. For *shudao*, the basic therapeutic tool is language and the psychotherapist plays a leading role in the therapy. Lu tries to mobilize the patients to fully exert their self-awareness and self-correction. He dwells on the self to seek both the causes of and solutions to mental distress, stressing a process of self-adaptation and correction. But one patient treated by Lu felt *shudao* to be intrusive and regulatory: "The treatment made me feel like my mind is in need of scrutiny and supervision by the doctor" (Lu 2006: 127).

While Lu stresses that *shudao* is a uniquely Chinese psychotherapy, his personality transformation theory is also a product of localizing Western psychotherapy. Like other Western psychotherapy, which focuses on the self, its core concepts include self-reflection and self-improvement.

Theories and methods of *shudao* are also derived from Confucian and Daoist precepts. For example, it requires a doctor to use *ren* (compassion) to "love" the patients, dredging the occlusion in them and inspiring them to have confidence to fight against mental distress. Similarly for patients, Lu teaches that if a person practices *ren* and observes *li* (rites of propriety), he or she will not suffer from anxiety, stress, or other psychological disorders and will enjoy health and longevity (*renzhe wu you; renzhe shou*). If people can effectively develop their own sense of compassion, they should be able to overcome all kinds of temptations and tribulations and gain peace of mind. In general, Lu (2006) considers compassion a cornerstone enabling doctors to support their clients and allowing clients with mental distress to reclaim the psychological balance that is key to mental and physical health (see also Hong 2016). However, he cautions that care must be taken not to overdo compassion as Confucius considered *ren* to be non-utilitarian. Since in reality too much emphasis on compassion may render people unrealistic, Lu cites Confucius's notion of *zhongyong*, "the Doctrine of Mean," a more stringent counterbalance to compassion, which prevents those who suffer from psychological disorders from being too subjective, obstinate, and delusional in their practice of *ren*. Drawing on both *ren* and *zhongyong*, *shudao* stresses self-moderation and self-cultivation for achieving mental health.

An example of the application of *ren* and *zhongyong* in *shudao* comes from one of my informants, a counselor named Jiang in Beijing (MKH-2012-d8). He indicated that the key to *shudao* therapy is to gain the client's trust so that the person can thoroughly proffer autobiographical accounts of perceived causes of his or her mental distress. To achieve ideal therapeutic efficacy, the counselor must be compassionate. Jiang offered one example. One of his clients, a middle-aged woman, works as a public servant at a government agency. By chance, she found out that her husband had had an affair with another woman. Fearing loss of "face," she did not tell anyone about her pain. However, such long-term suppressed pain and anger had a toll on her health. She finally had a nervous breakdown, suffering from insomnia, headache, night-mares, and absent-mindedness at work. She visited a doctor and took prescribed drugs, but the biomedical approach did not work for her. Finally, she went to see Jiang. Because of Jiang's warmth, patience, and empathy – being *ren* – this client finally confided to him in tears her long-subdued pain. Jiang not only attentively listened to her stories but also offered her advice on how to deal with negative feelings and even how to solve pragmatic issues like marital strife. He recommended through the use of *ren* and *zhongyong* that she forgive her husband and move on with life. Benefiting from this psychological dredging process and a balance of empathy and direction, this client not only became happier and more upbeat in a few months – that is, she developed a positive personality orientation rather than confronted social reality – her marital life also became blissful again. While *shudao* pays atten-tion to social causes of distress, ultimately what needs to be corrected is personality defects or "irrational" attitudes of the client. By essential-izing precepts of Confucianism, and integrating cognitive counseling techniques with the government interest in harmony, this counseling method appeals to clients from both the middle class and working class in the public sector as it is hospital-based and relatively more affordable than private counseling practices.

*Shudao* also draws on the Daoist notion of *wuwei*, literally "non-action," a central concept of Laozi's *Daodejing*. The notion of *wuwei* is multi-faceted and can include "not forcing," "acting spontaneously," and "flowing naturally with the moment." It is a concept used to explain *ziran*, the harmony with the *Dao* (the way the natural and social order operates). With this term, Laozi promoted simplicity and humility as key virtues, often in contrast to selfishness. These ideas also become the basis of *shudao*, which emphasizes letting "nature" take its course, letting things happen as they do. *Shudao* cites what Laozi taught people, not to pursue material things too much, as excessive prosperity will not last long, and strong and imperious people will not live long. These virtues and principles are important for one to maintain psychological balance and obtain peace of mind (Lu 2006). Moreover, these Daoist ideas instruct clients to *hutu* (pretend muddledness – a kind of smartness in the form of appearing muddled) – surviving by pretending not to know what is going on around them or "going with the flow." Clients should release their own agency and allow the counselor to lead and have all the control. In this sense, *shudao* constructs subjects who are not alienated by social contexts or immune to social wrongs but are moderate, obedient, and peaceful. They parallel or identify with the interests of the government, particularly for the purpose of social harmony and political stability.

*Imagery communication psychotherapy (ICP)*

While *shudao* emphasizes the role of language in cognitive reconstruction to help clients redress "patholological" thoughts or behaviors, ICP stresses the significance of images in transforming negative to positive feelings and healing clients. Professor Zhu Jianjun at Beijing Forestry University, who developed ICP in the 1990s, points out that the Chinese language is pictographic, with words stemming from meaningful pictures; the Chinese way of thinking thus tends to employ imagery and scenes to express feelings, desires, and thoughts.[4] This therapy has drawn attention mainly from other counselors, university students, and middle-class clients. Based on his view of typical Chinese characters, which tend to be sensitive, indirect, and reserved, Zhu uses ICP to help people return to their hearts to express themselves and find the meaning of self-existence. For Zhu, all psychological suffering is derived from lack of the sense of self-existence, misunderstanding one's self, or inappropriate responses to stress. Zhu contends that ICP is a way to talk to the heart, to see what the heart actually is and what it desires.

The ICP counseling procedures follow five stages. First is the introduction. The counselor explains the rules of imagination and counseling and asks the client to relax (ideally with eyes closed). Second comes imagination. The client is asked to enter into a contemplative state and search for an image intuitively. Guided meditation is sometimes adopted to inspire the client to find images that will form the basis of counseling. Therapists guide the client to imagine a particular image; the most frequently used one is a house. For Zhu, a house in the Chinese context symbolizes one's body or heart. He argues that clients may not be aware of the symbolic meanings of the house but in their subconsciousness they know what it represents. Another way to compel clients to find images for counseling is to imagine that they are walking downstairs in dim light. There is a mirror at the corner of the staircase, waiting for an image to emerge within it. That is what their minds look like. From there, the counselor begins to interact with the client about the view of his or her inner self. What does it say about him? What kind of person is she seeing? The third stage is analyzing and "embodied understanding" (tihui, understanding empathetically) of the images. The color, size, and location of the house in the client's imagination point to different psychological states or different types of distress. For example, if the house has a dark color, this often represents the client's negative feelings or attitudes. In the fourth stage, the counselor interacts with the client to understand his or her feelings, attitudes, and defense mechanisms and their transformations during the imagery analysis process. Finally, there is a brief summary and homework assignment. If the client imagines a dirty house during the counseling session, the counselor will give him or her homework like imagining cleaning the windows of the house every day.

Like *shudao* therapy, ICP also invokes Chinese tradition such as the precepts of Daoism and Buddhism, including the notion of *wuwei* (non-action, or acting without imposing) from the former and the notion of *buju buna* (rejectionlessness and detachment) from the latter, and applies these principles to the counseling process. Zhu argues that people are capable of perceiving the world and all experiences in their hearts without carrying out any cognitive activity. He offers one example. When one faces the sky at sunset, one may process information with symbols. However, sometimes one can completely forget all words and concepts, just letting the scene be reflected in the heart, where it arouses complex and indescribable feelings. Zhu thinks of this not as cognition but as a reflection, perception without processing information (Zhu 2008: 5). While Zhu does not invoke the notion of affect or emotion, which includes both cognition and bodily sensation (Ahmed 2004), he recognizes human experiences that go beyond cognition. The experience of going beyond cognition is the focus of ICP. Zhu thus instructs clients that they do not necessarily have to try to figure out all the meanings of each image.

One method in ICP to transform negative to positive images and attitudes about life is based on the Esoteric Buddhist practice of integrating the Buddha's image with oneself: that is, imagining the entrance of the Buddha's image into one's own body to acquire his wisdom and benevolence. In ICP, a client can choose a role model similar to him- or herself in terms of gender, stature, and other elements and acquire the desirable qualities of this person by imagining the integration of the two. (Zhu cautions that one should never choose an immoral or weak model for this task as the negative elements may also be acquired.) For

Zhu, this is a way of stimulating human subconsciousness, which contains enormous power, as physiological research has shown that only 15 percent of the human brain cells are utilized and the remaining 85 percent remain dormant (Zhu 2008).

Another way to transform negative images or attitudes to positive ones is through guided imagination. Zhu offers an example. A depressed client is imagining: "I am walking in the desert. No life around. I am walking without purpose but know what will happen: I will die and am not afraid." Zhu writes, the psychotherapist can support this client by saying: "Walk straight, and you will see hope. Many explorers found life under this circumstance. While this is the desert, there is still life here. If you look carefully, you will see insects and grasses" (Zhu 2008: 131). By offering positive images, counselors attempt to break down old vicious circles for clients who are pessimistic, negative, and lack love or support in their environments.

Similar to ICP is *huigui liaofa* (homecoming psychotherapy; hereafter *huigui*), the goals of which are to return to the self and heart. *Huigui* guides people to the ultimate paradise: the home of heart-spirits, pointing them to the ways to discover their true selves and to (re)gain inner peace. Also developed by Zhu Jianjun, along with co-founder Cao Yu, *huigui* asks clients to assess their lives according to a six-step cycle to find out what they worry most about, what they want, what measures they consider to satisfy their wants, what actions they actually take, what effects their actions generate, and how they explain what happens in their lives. According to Zhu, in the depths of their hearts, people need a sense of self-existence. *Huigui* is not about details of life but about its big picture and getting closer to the heart, thereby delving into the heart and subconsciousness more directly than other types of therapy (Zhu 2008).[5]

While Zhu Jianjun highlights the unique Chinese characteristics of his counseling theories and techniques by invoking the pictographic nature of Chinese thinking patterns and Buddhist and Daoist precepts, many of his clients, including psychotherapists, consider the interpretation of the meaning of images in ICP too contingent and the procedure as abstract as some Western counseling techniques. The interpretation of the images heavily relies on the psychotherapist's own ability to imagine and understand the relationship between an image and its (subconscious) psychological connotations for a client. Moreover, ICP counselors must be cautious in regulating clients' imaginations to prevent them invoking demonic images that may have harmful effects on their psychological health.

### "Giant infant" therapy

The famous Chinese counselor Wu Zhihong (2016) uses the concept of *juying* (giant infant, or adult infant) to explain social issues in China. The use of *juying* in therapy offers an alternative, more accessible approach to social and mental distress than Western inner child therapy. It starts with pragmatic social and individual issues and then traces them back to early infanthood, particularly the infant–mother relationships. Wu claims that Chinese psychological problems can be traced back earlier in infanthood than inner child therapy might suggest. He contends that 90 percent of social issues and most conflicts of love and hatred in China are due to stunted psychological development. Most Chinese, he claims, remain at the psychological level of an infant less than one year old, or, more specifically, not exceeding six months.[6] Three features characterize Wu's notion of *juying*: *gongsheng* (cohabitation), *quanneng zilian* (omnipotent narcissism), and *pianzhi fenlie* (schizoid bigotry).

Wu argues that at the core of Chinese culture, everyone wants to become a good infant and look for a good mother. The emotional tenor of most Chinese reflects this search for a mother. In adult life, this can lead to a choice of a marriage partner who resembles one's mother. Finding a mother serves two purposes: one is taken care of and one avoids facing the world alone (cohabitation); both, Wu believes, partly explain the collectivist foundations of Chinese culture.

In the desired state of cohabitation, *juying* claims, "I am my mother; my mother is mine. We are the same person; we share one body and the same psychological state. I know what you think without communicating with you; you know what I think without communicating with me." The *juying* considers her/himself the center of the world. Wu gives one example of the psychological consequences of cohabitation. Some Chinese tourists throw garbage when they travel. This, he argues, is because they consider themselves infants who cannot and do not want to take care of themselves. Rather, they need their mothers to look after them. Wu thus attributes the lack of ethical and moral discipline among Chinese tourists to their underdeveloped psychological state.

Another negative consequence of psychological cohabitation, according to Wu, is the risk of *gongsheng jiaosha* (cohabitation strangulation). Psychological cohabitation is a construction for a collective entity that requires unifying thoughts. Such unification of thought can kill individuality. Wu attributes strife and struggles between couples and among family members to this desire for ideological unification within a collective entity. One example Wu offers is the suicide of Yang Yuanyuan, a graduate student from Shanghai Maritime University whose mother had stayed with her since her undergraduate years, sleeping with her in one bed. Her own life was entirely consumed and strangled by her mother, who acted like an omnipotent empress.

Filled with omnipotent narcissism, *juying* declares, "I am God: the world turns around according to my will. If not, I will be enraged and can destroy the world." Wu exemplifies this narcissistic rage through the case of Han Lei. In a quarrel with a stranger regarding parking in Daxing, Beijing, on July 23, 2013, Han took this stranger's two-year-old baby from her stroller and threw her to the floor. The baby died three days later. Han was then sentenced to death. Wu suggests that

Han behaved like a *juying* performing his *quanneng zilian* (omnipotent narcissism): "If you violate my interest, I will destroy you."

The third characteristic of *juying* is *pianzhi fenlie* (schizoid bigotry), reflecting a clear-cut distinction between imagined good and bad, love and hatred. It is idealism without tolerance. Wu points out that such intolerance results in various manifestations of (public) retaliatory violence or crime in Chinese society. The infant behaves like a bigot: "My thought is correct; your thought is wrong. You must conform to my thought; otherwise, you have to die."

While *juying* have shortcomings and liabilities, Wu contends that their omnipotent narcissism should not be suppressed but needs to be understood, embraced, and channeled. It is argued that because of frustration Chinese experienced during infancy when they cohabited with their mothers, adults often develop as *juying*. These *juying* expect to become omnipotent gods. However, with needs unmet, they become omnipotent devils, who, once released, are destructive. Given this, the Chinese family, the exam-centered education system, and even the Chinese social hierarchy and culture are designed to suppress this potentially destructive force. Instead, however, Wu suggests that people release the narcissistic rage so that it can be humanized and relieved appropriately. *Juying* can become people with vigor and compassion. While Wu focuses on understanding, embracing, and channeling *juying* through talk-based counseling, other therapeutic techniques could also heal the inner child, for example dance therapy (see Chapter 3).

Wu also engages Confucianism by criticizing deeply rooted filial piety as a way of parental suppression through which parents act as giant infants to exploit children. Even though such a critique is confined to the interpersonal and intergenerational levels rather than going beyond the intersubjective realm to offer a critique of the broader political and economic process – the Chinese government's writing filial piety into the Constitution as a way of calling on the family to take care of the aging population rather than offer more public support – Wu's 2016 book, entitled *Juying Guo Nation of Giant Infants*, was banned in mid-February 2017. Chinese Internet users have speculated that Chinese censors banned the book because it is offensive to Chinese beliefs and traditions. This shows that Chinese counselors have the freedom to engage Confucian thought in psychotherapy, but criticizing Confucianism and its core concept of filial piety, which are instrumental to China's current governance, is not allowed.

Further, some Chinese counselors criticize the current focus on Western psychoanalytic obsessions as limited to pathogenic issues such as unconscious desires, the wounded inner child, and conflicts rooted in childhood experiences, by pointing out that a holistic and embodied perspective is more relevant to the Chinese context. Still, there has been a rapid surge in various versions of inner child therapy (*neizai xiaohai*, the core self with which one was born but that is damaged as the child adapts to social life) (Pritzker 2016). While therapists are aware of China's post-socialist transformation causing mental distress, it is often an unstated assumption. This framework highlights the absence of a caretaking and nurturing political or social system that is now replaced by impersonal and competitive market policies and politics that are alienating and engender pain and stress.


*Anger management*

While the above therapies tend to appeal to the middle class, the unique Chinese form of anger management mainly targets members of the working class as part of the state-sponsored psychotherapeutic intervention embedded in re-employment or poverty-relief programs, particularly for those who have been laid off from the public sector as a result of state enterprise restructuring. However, in general, although different counseling practices may target different classes of people in China, they share similar effects of addressing the person, not the circumstances.

While in China Western counseling for dealing with anger is available in diverse settings, here I want to focus on its particular iteration in a working-class community in Changping, as this counseling captures the alignment within contemporary psychological practice in China between self-interests and state interests (Yang 2016). Two philosophical traditions, Daoism and Confucianism, are often invoked in anger management in Changping (see Sundararajan 2015). Two components of anger, appraisal and display, are identified by counselors. The former deals with the reason for anger, the latter its expression. Confucian anger management focuses on anger display, while Daoism focuses on appraisal. Confucians accept the reason for one's anger and encourage "higher" (moral indignation) rather than "lower" (physical violence) expressions of the emotion. For them, social order is restored by *li* (ritual of propriety). *Li* dictates rules for both individual behavior and the social order. To adhere to *li*, one must restrain one's emotions and do what is right to conform to social norms for greater unity rather than giving in to passion or anger.

By contrast, Daoists seek to eliminate the reason for anger through cognitive reappraisal or a combination of purposeful neglect and nonjudgment (i.e., *hutu*). Daoist adherents commit themselves to psychosomatic purification (Komjathy 2014) from a variety of defilements of consciousness that may arise: "A person does not allow likes and dislikes to get in and do harm" (Zhuangzi, cited in Komjathy 2014: 120). To do this, they cultivate a kind of "emotionlessness" as the appropriate form of emotionality, rooted in stillness. Through stillness, one becomes free of entanglements such as reputation and social acceptance; one cultivates "true joy," "a state of spiritual freedom and bliss beyond the oscillations of gain and loss" (Komjathy 2014: 121).

In Changping, both these traditions affect the experience of anger and its management. Official anger-regulation strategies downplay sociopolitical factors that trigger anger, an approach that resonates more with Daoism. However, local authorities simultaneously turn to

Confucian notions of *chi* (shame or guilt), anger display, and self-cultivation when condemning "lower" forms of anger expression (i.e., physical violence).

Another anger management strategy is *nande hutu*, a combination of purposeful neglect, non-judgment, and cognitive reconstruction (see *shudao*). It originated in the thinking of Zheng Banqiao (1693–1765), a Qing dynasty official, philosopher, and artist from Jiangsu Province, whose ideas have regained popularity in China since the 1990s and have given rise to the popular practice of *hutuxue* (the study of muddledness). It means that while everyone wants smartness, real smartness, which is hard to achieve, is to be muddled. *Nande hutu* encompasses a kind of smartness that requires self-restraint (from getting angry).[7] More specifically, it expresses a Daoist precept which advocates putting appraisal (of causes of anger) on hold, a solution to anger similar to the no-judging approach in mindfulness. Muddledness aims to achieve an inner serenity and emotional equanimity anchored in the heart-mind (see Matthyssen 2012, 2015).

*Nande hutu* teaches people to take a broad look at life. It is mostly invoked to deal with (negative) emotions such as anger, frustration, angst, powerlessness, resentment, and disappointment. As a way of self-cultivation deeply concerned with social morality, *nande hutu* carries the promise of increasing moral virtue, psychological well-being, and wisdom. This can hardly be perceived as a passive state but is a proactive approach to dealing with stressors (see Cheng et al. 2010). With the harmonization of mind and body and through individual self-cultivation, *nande hutu* contributes to achieving harmony on different levels and even offers opportunities for active personal growth (Confucianism).

The practice of *nande hutu* is mindful; one seeks to distance oneself from negative feelings and focus on something tolerable and positive in order to avoid anger and moral indignation. It is a mode of secondary control consisting of "attempts to change one's thoughts or behavior to fit the environment" (Cheng et al. 2010: 403). It differs from primary control, which refers to efforts made in an attempt to change external or environmental factors to fit one's needs and expectations. While only a few studies have applied mindfulness to the treatment of anger problems (Vannoy and Hoyt 2004), scholars suggest that mindfulness-based interventions may be ideal for the management of anger, since they focus on tolerance of negative emotional states, reduction of emotional reactivity, and the incompatibility of mindfulness and angry rumination (Wright et al. 2009).

*Nande hutu* reminds people of the necessity to detach themselves from anger and pretend to be muddled about the consequences of social change and injustice. However, today anger is both an effect of and a response to widespread sociopolitical transformations. In *nande hutu*, these sociopolitical causes of people's anger go unarticulated. The wisdom of acting *hutu* to distance oneself from the hardship and social injustice one experiences individualizes and moralizes anger, thereby rendering people immune to social critique.

*Folk and faith healing*

Scholars have reported abuses by indigenous healers in China and been critical about the lack of efficacy of traditional forms of healing for serious illnesses (Li and Phillips 1990). Yet Arthur Kleinman (1995) was impressed that the structures of traditional healing centered on human experience and its modes of interaction give these practitioners a way of reaching others. They may be less advantaged in technology but more advantaged in humanity.

Mental health in Zhangqiu has been understood by some people as a consequence of demonic or spirit possession. Some of my informants, including local officials, turned to folk healers for relief from their distress. One of my informants, a woman named Hao whom I met at ZYH, had suffered phobia (ZYH-2013-p2). The direct trigger of her phobia was when someone knocked at her windows one night when her husband was not at home. She was so scared that she could not sleep for a whole week and dressed herself in thick winter clothes even in the hot summer. Since then she had refused to open her windows or interact with others. Her husband took her to ZYH and got medication for her symptoms, but because of the heavy side-effects and her concerns about drug addiction, she stopped taking this. Her husband also took her to Beijing for psychotherapeutic treatment through, for example, EMDR (eye movement desensitization and reprocessing)[8] and CBT; however, none of these therapies worked on her as she had no resources to follow through for long-term multiple counseling in Beijing. Finally, her sister took her to see a Buddhist master in Zhangqiu, who eventually converted her to Buddhism. Gradually her fear and insomnia disappeared and she opened herself to the world again. Hao told me about her faith in Buddha and the sense of security and peace she felt from believing in Buddha through meditation and chanting *xinjing* (the heart sutra), which has become popular as a resource of self-cultivation and healing in China. These practices helped her overcome the fear and insecurity she had experienced since the triggering event. To me, her faith in Buddha works on her phobia by reconstructing her cognition – the source of security and peace derived from invoking the image of Buddha and the heart sutra. This form of healing resembles CBT but goes beyond it by incorporating bodily and affective dimensions (see also Chapter 2 on how prayers heal "Internet addiction").

## CONCLUSION

The recent rise of psychological counseling and its diverse origins and applications in China have ushered in a new or revitalized body of therapeutic expertise with new practices of therapy, new ways of construing, evaluating, and actualizing social relations, and new ways of exploring spaces of interiority, thereby creating new sites of defiance and resistance. The emphasis on the self, interiority, and *xinli hua* (reasoning from and to the heart) further contributes to and reinforces the rise of individual-centered ethics, which resonates with the government's call for individuals to be responsible for their own difficulties and lives. There is an emerging inner revolution in China. The turn to notions of the heart, subconsciousness, or the inner child for salvation and solutions ultimately enacts neoliberal ideology that stresses individual autonomy, which, however, does not entirely suit the historical and cultural specificity of China, a country still in the process of transitioning from collective socialist ethics to individualistic ethics correlating with a market-based economy.

The hybridizing of indigenous and Western forms of knowledge and behavior as is unfolding in China has hegemonic effects. Such hybridity encourages people to believe they are subjecting themselves to indigenous Chinese healing resources while these methods actually graft elements of Chinese cultural tradition onto Western ideologies of psychotherapy to holistically mobilize the inner force of individuals for relief and salvation, penetrating their hearts and minds more thoroughly and more profoundly than Western psychotherapy. The deployment of Chinese cultural traditions in psychotherapies not only de-medicalizes counseling but also popularizes psychology as part of everyday ethics and everyday practice. Instead of flattening counseling psychology through the medical model in terms of health and illness, the hybrid counseling methods practiced in China integrate counseling with the Chinese tradition of self-cultivation and life-nurturing. The emphasis on Chinese cultural and historical specificity and everyday life as resources for psychological relief illustrates a trend of psychologization, which renders therapeutic governing banal while endowing therapeutic practices with cultural sensitivity and depth and creating an impression of facilitating self-realization and maturity. However, these impressions mask the hegemony behind the counseling adaptations and conceal the potential for penetration of state interests into the individual mind and heart.

# 7 | Happiness and Psychological Self-Help _____

We have nothing, but *xiao que xing* [small but certain happiness].
*A laid-off worker in Changping, Beijing*

For he who is really *ren* [compassionate] is never unhappy; he who is really
wise is never perplexed; and he who is really brave is never afraid.
*Confucius*, Analects *(13:30)*

Happiness comes from the heart, not from the environment.
*A Chinese folk saying*

A Zhangqiu official charged with writing the city's history once showed
me an article published in *Lingdao Wencui* (Leaders' Digest) (Gu 2013)
entitled "God Can Only Help You Find the Wound," which he thought
was relevant to my research on therapeutic governance. The article told
the story of how physical suffering had shaped the character of late
Venezuelan President Hugo Chávez. According to the article, after an
accident at age seven, Chávez suffered so much pain that he considered
suicide. His grandfather took him to the local hospital, where doctors
found a steel needle piercing his chest. They were able to remove the
object, but Chávez continued to suffer lingering pain. He was frustrated and disillusioned, complaining to his grandfather that the God-
like physicians had failed – they were able to locate his wound, but
unable to end his pain. His grandfather replied by showing Chávez his
own leg, in which a bullet had been deeply embedded during the

country's earlier civil war. Doctors had once offered to take the bullet out, but at the risk of costing him his leg. He had declined surgery in order to continue to walk on his own. Chávez's grandfather concluded that God can only help you find the wound; you must heal yourself with confidence, perseverance, and stamina. To become a true man, you must develop a persistent heart, battling pain, like fighting an enemy on the battlefield. Chávez took this message to heart, and applied it to catapult his meteoric ascent to power.

I agreed with my informant that this story exemplifies an area of my work. I would categorize it as part of the genre of *xinling jitang* (chicken soup for the soul) (Yu 2006; Y. Zhang 2014), which has been crucial to the exploding self-help movement in China. "Chicken soup" literature, encompassing elements from success studies, psychology, and religion, highlights the significance of one's *xinnian* (faith) in helping and healing oneself. Like other stories in this genre, which tend to hide the complex, multi-faceted factors that contribute to success, the Chávez story sensationalizes one element of his success: his belief in himself, his stamina and perseverance. This element is then promoted to a "truth" that can be applied as common sense. Key words highlighted in *xinling jitang* include *renrang* (tolerance), *nuli* (diligence), *xinnian* (belief or faith), *zhizu* (contentment), and *gan'en* (gratitude) (Luo 2016). Such strategic reduction makes the narration sensational, appealing, and inspirational. The Chávez story also parallels a theme in China's therapeutic governance: God-like government-therapists can only identify social wounds or individual problems. If the state attempts to entirely resolve problems, this can bring ruin to the whole system. Individuals must pick up where the state leaves off, have faith in themselves, and, like Chávez and his grandfather, develop stamina and perseverance to endure or resolve problems on their own.

With the gradual collapse of socialist-era work units and people's communes in China since the 1980s, a new desire for individual freedom has arisen in such areas as love, marriage, career, and family, which are no longer politically scrutinized or regulated. It is now legitimate for individuals to pay attention to their personal lives. It is in this context that *xinling jitang*, which addresses private and inner lives, has emerged. With privatization and economic restructuring since the mid-1990s, the government has also stressed economic development and social stability, and *xinling jitang*, alongside its function in relieving emotional, psychological, and social disorders, serves these government goals. I contend that, as part of China's psychoboom, *xinling jitang* captures psychology's "overflow" into the broader realms of society and its entanglement with power mechanisms. I pay particular attention to how *xinling jitang* is co-opted via state-led happiness campaigns and the official promotion of *zheng nengliang* (positive energy) for achieving social, economic, and political objectives and cultivating happy, productive, and moral subjects.

## HISTORY AND SCOPE OF CHINESE SELF-HELP

China's self-help movement has roots in its American counterpart. Many of the country's bestselling self-help books are actually translations of US publications. Napoleon Hill's *Think and Grow Rich* (1937/1953) described the use of repeated positive thought to attract happiness and wealth by tapping into an infinite intelligence. The basic structure of these books is, first, a suggestion that there is a flaw in people because of the culture that guides or programs them, and, second, a suggestion of what might be done to correct this problem. That is, self-help books offer both a critique of the culture and a solution to it (Dolby 2005: 4–5). Yet the books actually maintain the stability of culture, ensuring that some elements of it go unquestioned and are therefore preserved (Dolby 2005: 11). The US self-help movement has since grown vast and varied, serving the desire of an American audience that supports self-awareness, self-reliance, and self-education (Dolby 2005: xii). In China, meanwhile, self-help genres (particularly for women) also flourished early – starting in the 1920s after the May Fourth Movement. For example, in the journal *Xin Nüxing* (New Women), Xia Mianzun (1886–1946), an accomplished educator and translator, offered advice particularly for women. He argued that bitterness or happiness was determined not by the external environment, but by one's heart-attitude. Xia advocated a shift in women's heart-attitude: if women could just think of their status as being greater than men's because they produce babies and fulfill glorious, sanctifying wifely duties, they would naturally demand acknowledgment of their value from society. It is only because women lack self-awareness of their own value that they are relegated to a degraded status: "Since you have to be busy, do not humiliate yourself in your busyness. Instead, you should exert yourselves, realize yourselves and highlight your advantages, so that you can make the nation, society, and, your rival men to recognize and appreciate your value and status through your busyness" (Xia 1926: 67).

Xia's work captures the ways that Chinese self-help has diverged from the US tradition: it is a hybrid, combining the "Western" notion of the psyche or mind with a uniquely Chinese emphasis on the heart. In *xinling jitang*, the heart is portrayed as divided: one half is clear-minded, the other murky and tolerant of injustice in order to be at peace with the social world. Over time, this has caused some people in China to turn against self-help, while in the United States, self-help has largely escaped such a backlash. Today, widespread anti-*xinling jitang* sentiment finds expression through Chinese microblogging (*weibo*). Bloggers argue that the genre is reductive, that it numbs readers and immunizes them against social critique. Worse yet, they say that the literature does not benefit readers, as the self-help audience actually becomes more sensitive to stress, and can manifest more depressive symptoms than those who do not engage with it.[1] They argue that self-help is a way of "feeding oneself by drawing a pancake" (*hua bing chong ji*); it offers people illusions and draws them into an enclosed bubble of self-reflection without considering broader social and political processes.

Yet the birth of *xinling jitang* in China responded to a set of social and historical changes. One of these was China's "belief crisis" (*xinyang weiji*), which derived from a public and academic debate that began in the 1980s as a result of relaxed political control. People began to ask what core beliefs they collectively held, and no easy answers emerged. Arguably, this crisis had already been lurking within the monopoly of political ideology in people's ethical lives in Mao's era, when the most valued aspect of the self was moral character. Character safeguarded against a life of sloth, disloyalty, and ideological degeneracy. Character and moral integrity could be built through loyalty to Chairman Mao, self-discipline, political studies, and hard work. When China launched economic reform in the late 1970s and these strong, state-deployed edicts began to weaken, what resulted was a void of belief and a psychological and moral "vacuum" because of the decline of people's acceptance of Communism and the releasing of market forces (Bell 2008).

In the post-Mao reform era, personality has been reconceived as the sum of personal qualities that cause one to be liked by others or to stand out in a crowd (cf. Cushman 1992), and there is far less stress on character or moral integrity. The concern for developing personality resembles the kind of think-properly-and-grow-rich program in American mesmerism (Meyer 1980; Cushman 1992), making psychological techniques an accessible way to power and fame. Psychology provides a new terrain for enhancement and productivity.

Today, there are at least three major trends of psychological self-help in China. First, there is online counseling offered by professional psychotherapists, such as those on the well-known daily show *Xinli Fangtan* (Psychology Talk Show) on China Central Television (CCTV), which moves talk therapy from private counseling rooms to public screens, making confessing one's personal problems a subject of mass entertainment (cf. Illouz 2008). Second, problem-oriented genres offer pragmatic advice or solutions to specific problems, including anxiety, anger issues, marital problems, and procrastination. And finally, growth-oriented genres advocate positive and encouraging messages about life and happiness. This last dimension of self-help is also called *xinling chengzhang* – roughly, heart-spirit growth, which does not focus on problems or pathology, but rather on nurturing positive potential – and includes "third force" (*di san shili*) psychological self-help. "Third force" addresses an ambivalent "third state" between health and illness, or subhealth, which, as noted in the Introduction, impacts a vast majority of China's population.

These trends in *xinling jitang* exist in the context of greater recognition of medically defined distress in China. Some 190 million Chinese reportedly suffer mental disorders, including anxiety, substance abuse, and mild to severe psychiatric illnesses (Shao 2016). However, as mentioned in the Introduction, psychological professionals in China are not sufficient to meet the needs of mental health care. In this context, psychological self-help becomes imperative to help people cope with psychological distress on their own. *Xinling jitang* helps address a dilemma in China's mental health care: on the one hand, hospital-based psychiatric treatment is socially recognized but highly stigmatized; on the other hand, improving the field's reputation entails both removing public stigmas against mental illness and providing opportune resources for treating those who are experiencing psychological distresses. While (new) institutional initiatives attempt to popularize the field of mental health, they also inject new meanings into the therapeutic framework, which gradually shifts the focus from severe psychiatric disorders to everyday distress, manifesting in the current rise of (online) counseling and the self-help movement in China. The kind of counseling offered in Chinese hospitals is predominated by a medical model with abstract concepts and heavily therapeutic language (Clay 2002; Han and Zhang 2007); such a medicalized model imbued with pathologized language deters people from seeking healing from counselors, given the strong stigma associated with mental illness in China. On the flipside, self-help allows people to self-heal and gain psychological insights without risking their social status or "face."

Meanwhile, rampant consumerism in China has nurtured the growth of *xinling jitang*. Members of the middle class are interested in reading books about individual development and career advancement (Wang 2014; Zhang 2015; see also Farquhar 2001) and are the largest users and consumers of the *xinling jitang* genre. In a survey that asked respondents what genres of books they read frequently, about 32 percent identified self-help and personal development as their most-read genres (Wang 2014: 6) in order to survive and succeed, particularly in an environment of increasing competition.

The self-help genre also includes books on the teachings of Confucius and other ancient Chinese schools of thought (see Y. Zhang 2014 on Confucianism; Zhang 2015 on Buddhism and Daoism), especially those offering practical advice for work and life. One such bestseller is Yu Dan's (2006) book on Confucianism, over 10 million copies of which have been sold throughout China.[2] The success of Yu's book is attributed to its simple, positive, and apolitical nature and its stories about interpersonal relationships, self-awareness, and the pursuit of happiness. Her success shows that the middle class prefers its personal development advice wrapped in traditional Chinese virtue (Wang 2014: 6). Meanwhile, Yu has also received immense criticism from both the public and scholars for her vulgarization and psychologization of Confucius's *Analects*, which implicitly serves the government's interests, including social stability. She has even been called a "heart-spirit terrorist" and the kind of *xinling jitang* she delivers has been castigated as "heart-spirit arsenic." Her famous *jitang* example includes her remarks on China's smog: "Close the doors and windows so as not to allow the smog into your room; then turn on your air purifier so as not to allow the smog into your lungs. If this does not work, you have to rely on your spiritual protection to prevent smog getting into your heart." Her pattern of *jitang* is exemplified by her sayings such as "No matter how ugly this world is, I persist in the beautifying of my heart," and "Even if you raped my body, you cannot rape my spirit or tarnish my heart-soul." Famous cultural critic Wang Xiaoyu states that "Yu Dan is an advanced version of Lei Feng.[3] Both are spiritual atom bombs, playing the role of *jingshen weiwen* [spiritually sustaining stability]. … For Yu Dan, people's complaints about smog and society all derive from their own hearts not being peaceful enough, their self-cultivation not being intense enough, and their heart-souls not expansive enough" (Wang Xiaoyu 2016). Many commentators view Yu Dan's interpretation of Confucianism as fulfilling political objectives. In their view, her calls for people "to be content," to "always find the problem within oneself," and to "be grateful to be alive" not only numb and placate people but also obscure the distinction between right and wrong.

Finally, the self-help movement has been highly gendered from the time Xia Mianzun was writing in the 1920s and remains so today. In Beijing bookstores and newsstands, self-help literature is often found next to women's books and magazines. The formulas in many of these books target women. Women are encouraged to be nurturing and flexible in their marriage, for example. Wang Xiaoxing, a housewife and author of bestselling cooking books, who has been celebrated by the All-China Women's Federation, compares women to potatoes because they perform flexible femininity, acting not only as impressive garnish but also as soft "mashed" accompaniments. Men, she claims, resemble noodles: no matter what kind of dressing you put on them, they are essentially the same. Women should not try to change their husbands, but rather perform flexible domestic femininity – mash themselves (Yu 2011). Of course, the formulae dictating the gendered self-help literature about women and their roles as "wise mothers and virtuous wives" are often created by and serve the interests of men (cf. Friedan 1965). The values and gender ideologies imbued in *xinling jitang* are male-oriented.

## HAPPINESS AS THERAPY, SELF-MANAGEMENT, AND SELF-ADVANCEMENT

Dozens of programs and series on the country-wide state-sponsored CCTV, as well as on local cable TV, frequently use terms like *xingfu, kuaile, huanle,* or *kaixin,* all of which is roughly translated as happiness. This is no accident, but rather part of a larger marketing strategy of the Party-governed media to promote happiness as the ultimate goal in life. This strategy, in place since 2006, has several aims, including stimulating consumption. More generally, happiness has become an index to evaluate economic growth and a means of governing efficiency, particularly in relation to the project of achieving a "harmonious society," ongoing since 2004. Put simply, happiness sustains social harmony (see Yang 2014; Zhang 2015).

In fact, since the mid-1990s, Chinese people, especially those from underprivileged groups, have become less happy. Widespread socioeconomic dislocation has degraded living conditions for millions. This has led to a weakening of the Communist Party's eudaemonic legitimacy – the justification of its rule through efficient provision of economic benefits to individuals (Chen 1994). Happiness promotion among marginalized groups has become a form of governance that, operating in a therapeutic mode, seeks to reassert control by the Party. As mentioned, women in particular (and especially those from underprivileged groups) are mobilized by media and arms of the state to play a key role in disseminating happiness. This occurs through, for example, the work of *peiliao* (chatting companions), who are mainly laid-off women workers or rural migrant women trained in preliminary psychology or counseling techniques to perform informal counseling and transmit happiness in their capacity as housewives or domestic workers (J. Yang 2015).

Happiness campaigns overlap with and support the self-help movement. Happiness is promoted by Chinese psychological gurus or counselors as a way of self-regulation and self-management. Zhang Defen

(2016), a Taiwanese guru whose books have become immensely popular in mainland China, states that true happiness comes from one's inner self rather than from the external world. She contends that neither success nor money or power can make one happy. Everyone is given a life script, which is actually not important; what matters is how one performs based on that script. She advises people to make happiness their first priority, to make up their minds to be happy, and constantly remind themselves to stay happy. She suggests that one should try to stay close to one's self, to one's inner child. To comfort or heal one's wounded inner child, who does not feel loved, approved, or secure, and to obtain happiness, Zhang proposes three steps. First, we should slow the breath, as breath can be used to comfort our inner child. When we focus on our breath, we stay close to ourselves and experience the here and now, our inner being. Second, we should relax the body to see which body part is tense, and then relax it consciously with breathing. Finally, we should relax the nerves of the brain and empty the mind: when we make up our mind to be happy, we use the power of our mind strategically to control our behavior. In general, for Zhang, happiness is internal. It can be performed and cultivated through breathing, relaxing, and staying close to one's inner being. Before Zhang turned to her way of promoting happiness in China, she gave an example of the kind of happiness advocated in Bhutan, where the king does not allow foreign businesses into the country in order to make sure the people continue to enjoy relatively organic communities and a carefree, slow-tempo lifestyle. Her emphasis on the role of the self and the turn to one's internal life in cultivating happiness constitutes an implicit criticism of the Chinese government's failure to protect its people from the stress triggered by a sea change as a result of widespread socioeconomic dislocation and the country's integration into the global economy.

One of the political effects of current happiness campaigns in China is the inculcation of new values such as self-care, self-realization, and self-enterprise. The emphasis on the self as the source of happiness constitutes a critique of the Maoist ideology that held that happiness derived from politics and from the elevation of the collective over the individual (McGrath 2009). Self-cultivation has been key to Chinese personhood and Confucian culture. However, what the self is and how to cultivate it in the Chinese context needs to be defined. The self is located in and derived from the interpersonal field, including interpersonal interactions and the larger sociohistorical sphere of cultural values and beliefs. However, in Zhang Defen's happiness promotions and other self-focused psychotherapies, the intrapsychic emphasis diverts responsibility for individuals from socioeconomic arrangements and places it on the self-contained individual.

### "Little happiness in hand" and "fake happiness"

One strand of happiness-oriented self-help is embodied in the popularity of various sayings or aphorisms about the keys to happiness. One of these sayings as noted in the opening epigraph of this chapter, is *xiao que xing*, translated as "small but certain happiness" or "little happiness in hand." Coined by the Japanese writer Haruki Murakami, the saying has been widely circulated in Chinese media, happiness campaigns, and everyday discourse, particularly among the working class. *Xiao que xing* refers to the ephemeral but happy moments in life that result from small things, the daily details of existence to which everyone has access (Cui 2011) – like hearing the voice of a friend over the phone or realizing while standing in line that the line is moving quickly. In Changping, where I have done research since 2002, the term *qiong huanle* (being poor but enjoying life) conveys a similar meaning. For underemployed workers in Changping, the meager income from manual labor or taxi-driving cannot sustain a decent life. But people try to make the best of it, by enjoying themselves and their solidarity with former co-workers and neighbors. They play poker together in the evenings when they do not need to go out for extra work. They share secret tips on how to save water in order to slow down the water meter, which could trick water-meter-reading officers. They also share tips, exclusively with one another, on where to buy cheap vegetables, and where to fetch mineral spring water free of charge, rather than buying bottled water. By highlighting optimism despite hardship, the notions of *xiao que xing* and *qiong huanle* constitute survival strategies for these workers.

Meanwhile, in Changping, the workers' practice of *qiong huanle* was also a carnivalesque strategy to express grievances or anger because of their downward mobility and the devastating living conditions resulting from mass layoffs. In the wake of the SARS outbreak in May 2003, over 300 taxi-drivers (most of them re-employed laid-off workers) took over the streets of Changping, blocking traffic in front of the district government for three days in order to pressure the government to regulate the taxi industry and create more jobs. Because of the panic constructed by the media during the disease outbreak, people seldom went outside. Taxi-drivers had no business, and the situation did not change much when the health epidemic was contained. Instead of staying idle, the drivers organized a strike and broke the spell of fear. Many took comfort in their numbers and said they were unafraid. They were laughing, joking, playing poker, or listening to music; they made noise by whistling and honking their horns. They had the self-comforting attitude of being *qiong huanle*; for them, the best response to the state-led anti-working-class policy is to live happily and healthily.

*Qiong huanle* resembles the Confucian notion of *le*, often translated as "joy," referring to the acceptance of adverse circumstances in terms of the absence of worry and anxiety. *Le* emphasizes not a state of emotional exhilaration, but rather a state of moving along at ease with the flow of things, calmly and smoothly (see Shun 2011). However, while workers claimed to practice *qiong huanle* to downplay their political motivation, their organized protests showed that through such collective challenge to authorities, they aimed at ultimately achieving something for their own benefit. Their deployment of the genre of *qiong huanle* was to remove the burden of anxiety and fear of repression. By using laughter and noise as weapons with which to confront authority, participants were emboldened to engage in acts of insubordination (see also Flam 2004). Yet while their collective action helped them feel less fearful, protesters tried to avoid extreme actions that might provoke the hostility of the police and government. Nor did organizers really expect any concrete resolution. Rather they felt that open and collective displays of anger could at least serve as a wake-up call for the government to become aware of workers' economic difficulties and the kind of power those workers could muster if there were no changes in the desired direction. Useful in justice when treated as substantive and deserving of attention, anger can yield a sense of liberation (Lyman 2004), but it must first find a critical voice. Practices like *qiong huanle* may partially help workers achieve this.

A cousin of both *xiao que xing* and *qiong huanle* is *wei xingfu*, or fake happiness. *Wei xingfu* refers to the kind of happiness that is lower than the average living standard enjoyed by ordinary people. It particularly targets members of underprivileged groups in programs that purportedly show people how to reconstruct happiness after their previous satisfaction with life has been destroyed by privatization (see Yang 2013). A typical joke about happiness promotion in China is reflected in the following widely circulated folk report of a conversation:

*Journalist*: Are you happy?
*Peasant*:   Yes. I am.
*Journalist*: What are you happy about?
*Peasant*:   I don't know.

The exchange captures a kind of solicited happiness that is a product of happiness promotions and the harmonious society propaganda, especially among marginalized groups. Chinese commentator Han Haoyue (2010) contends that the kind of happiness of members of disadvantaged groups represented in the media is actually *wei xingfu* (false or fake happiness). It differs significantly from the generally accepted ideal of happiness: it represents a lower standard of positive feeling and contentment in the name of happiness, a level below even that afforded by the average Chinese standard of living. Happiness that occurs in a passive relation to whatever one is given and whatever forces control one's fate is self-deceiving. It romanticizes pain and suffering as hope and potential. Such happiness promotion apparently satisfies contingent needs, interests, and aspirations of the government, the managerial class or the middle class. However, it also attracts contestation, especially from marginalized groups (Yang 2013).

*Therapeutic consumption*

Happiness both arises from and advances consumption. In the realm of self-help, commodities and their advertisements are imbued with psychological precepts. Consumers buy these commodities in the belief that they will help them relieve stress and achieve happiness and self-fulfillment. We can call this therapeutic consumption. Commodities become transforming objects. The self identifies with the happiness and lifestyles of models/celebrities in the advertisements, whose qualities are attached to the objects: for example, the happy housewives in many advertisements in self-help media in China (cf. Ewen 1989; Cushman 1992). The idea is that people will become happy and confident through consuming these objects and services.

Psychology is used by business to boost consumption. Consuming is like relating: it is satisfying, soothing, and energizing; it drives away loneliness and makes life rich and rewarding. Consuming is often portrayed in this way in contemporary advertising. Offering optimism and pragmatism, psychology plays a key role in the realm of business.

Advertising attempts to mimic the ideology of therapy. Advertisements associate the product with happy, clean, vigorous models and imaginary states of being, addressing the worries of uncertain and confused individuals who are searching for a way to reintegrate their sense of selfhood (cf. Cushman 1992). Individuals who have been addicted to a drug often describe their relationship with the drug in a similar way. For instance, drugs – the consumer item – are powerful forces in the addict's life. When consumers are addicted, the commodity has complete control over them. It is the irresistible object. The consumer item, used to fill the consumer up, takes on a life of its own. In this sense, the commodity has become the ultimate transformative device: it can even completely remake identity (Norwood 1985; Bartlett 2016).

### Zheng nengliang (*positive energy*)

Happiness and *xinling jitang* genres in China are imbued with *zheng nengliang* (positive energy). For example, Yu Dan has been widely ridiculed by Chinese Internet commentators as having "her whole body filled with *zheng nengliang* and her blood saturated with *jitang.*" *Zheng nengliang* means both "being positive" and "political correctness." Since the 1980s, the term *zheng nengliang* has entered into the Chinese discourse amidst the psychoboom and the advent of positive psychology. From official propaganda to folk commentary, people promote positive energy, advocating and disseminating *zheng nengliang*. People today are compelled to socialize with others who have positive rather than negative energy. If you are full of positive energy, it seems, that energy is a kind of contagion, improving the positive energy level of those surrounding you. This positive energy does not seem troubled by a society marked by rampant corruption or hidden rules (*qian guize*) (see Chapter 1). Rather, the official promotion of positive energy, correlating with its folk support, has rendered it a kind of opiate that facilitates shirking away from social reality. Using positive energy to fill the "vacuum" created by a lack of social morale is reminiscent of religious belief that encourages those who live at the bottom of a social hierarchy to expect happiness in the next world and ignore their current miserable circumstances. Indeed, the discourse of *zheng nengliang* tends to invoke precepts of Buddhism (finding happiness in "the next world"). Unlike Confucianism, which usually leads to restriction and exclusiveness, Buddhism points to openness and tolerance. This partly explains why Buddhism has become the choice for Chinese people from all walks of life for spiritual guidance and psychological solace.

One example of the official promotion of positive energy is propaganda surrounding a beggar from Zhaoyuan, Shandong Province, who, while making a living by collecting garbage, donates all his savings to help poor kids go to school. People find the story moving, but it is rare to hear people ask why students should require donations from a garbage collector to attend school (Lin Zuxian 2016). How is tax money being spent? To a great extent, the discourse of positive energy through official media sings the praises of the government's achievements and upholds social morals that conform to official policies and ideologies. However, as commentators contend, if there is no substantial social reform, no matter how much positive energy the government promotes and instills, it cannot transform a demoralized society marked by intensified inequality and social stratification. Thus, positive energy as a subliminal psychological discourse and a dose of spiritually numbing medicine attempts to fool the masses and mask the inadequacy of social services and policy failures.

## TRANSFORMING CONFUCIANISM INTO *XINLING JITANG*

As mentioned, the brand of self-help called *di san shili* (third force), which has emerged roughly since 2006 (Wang 2008; Zheng 2009), addresses subhealth. But third force also addresses a general acknowledged lack of individuals' "psychological quality" and the increasing loss of morals in Chinese society (see Yang 2017). Instead of introducing brand-new methods, third force optimizes pragmatic methods of counseling and precepts of social work. Third force trainers see psychological disorder not as pathology, but as an opportunity to strengthen people who are destined and prepared to undertake important tasks. For this reason, psychologists advocating third force often call it *qiangzhe xinlixue* (superman psychology). Writ large, third force aims to construct deeper psychological and moral mechanisms to help people cope with change. Like other strands of self-help, this goal parallels state interests, particularly in social stabilization and market advancement.

Here I focus on one genre of third force that draws on Confucian virtue ethics to relieve social, moral, and psychological disorders. These Confucian ethics tend to humanize and moralize both market competition and the often crippling effects of economic restructuring. Third force psychological training is hybrid, flexible, personable, and performative, combining the interpretation of Confucian doctrines with metaphors, fables, and personal stories. Such training putatively focuses on the trainee, not the trainer. One of its key features is *gan ran li*, or "affectivity." For instance, at a training session at a university auditorium in Beijing in summer 2012, the trainer, a professor of social work and Marxism, asked the trainees to use their hands and mouths to create the climatic atmosphere of rain, as rain in Chinese culture points to abundance and wealth. To create the effect of pouring rain – symbolizing a windfall of good fortune – one needs to use not only one's hands and mouth, but also one's feet, the trainer explained. Thus, the strength of the whole body is required to achieve a windfall. Through such embodied exercises, the trainer demonstrated that the degree of one's success relies on the degree of one's dedication and effort, amplifying the significance of individual efforts in one's success while sidelining social, economic, and political factors in that trajectory.

Probably the most exaggerated affective prelude for third force training was one of the sessions offered by *chuangzao fengsheng* (Creating Abundance – a private psychological training center) (Luo 2016). The trainer shouted, "If all 20 million Beijingers got up in the morning, thinking they could feel the sunshine and that the air was good, there could be no smog in Beijing. This is called *gongzhen* [co-palpitation]." This trainer then asked the trainees to "wave your wings and participate in the co-palpitation," which allegedly could open the passage of energy between their hearts and the universe. This passage, he claimed, could solve various problems in their careers, marriages, and families, and bring about happiness and success. How does this mystical passage open up? The answer is to pay expensive training fees (ranging from 50,000 to 800,000 RMB) for more learning in "Creating Abundance" (Luo 2016). Such an affective prelude to the *xinling jitang* style of psychological training not only compels the participants to directly enter the atmosphere of the training, but also allows them to have a taste of the efficacy of the message delivered by the guru.

The popularization or vulgarization of Confucianism in this strand of third force self-help opens up (new) space to further commercialize and moralize psychology, which intensifies the regulation of individual lives and constitutes a more hegemonic form of psychologization, as it focuses on everyday life, regulating individuals' routine behaviors. On the cover of a pamphlet I received while attending a training session in summer 2009 were the following words: "Confucius' *Analects* conveys a simple and warm attitude toward life. It teaches us how to enjoy happiness in our soul, how to adapt to daily order, and find our own compass in life."

Such psychological training adopts a moralizing model; it claims that the psychological imbalance or disorders people encounter in the age of change and market competition are ultimately caused by moral or ethical failures, especially according to Confucian ethics. That is, psychological health is derived from individual ethical and moral choice and behavior. Its main purpose is not to transmit knowledge but to direct people's conduct. Such moral psychology based on Confucian ethics sets out to criticize the negative consequences of market competition and socioeconomic dislocation, but in fact its emphasis on success coincides with neoliberal entrepreneurship, and its promotion of benevolence, mutual assistance, and social harmony facilitates the Party's interest in social stabilization. Its advocacy of filial piety and social hierarchy, moreover, sustains the existing power structure.

This self-help genre treats psychological problems as caused not by social inequality, but by lack of proper psychological mechanisms, which can be obtained through proper training. The genre stresses participation in a certain activity and interaction with one another in a group setting, but does not consider the macrosocial, economic, and political context that contributes to the person's problems, nor does it take into account the individual's class, gender, and other elements of his or her identity by invoking "A gentleman's anxieties concern *dao*; he has no anxiety concerning poverty" (*Analects* 15:31). This moralization of social and psychological problems not only echoes the governing principle proposed by former President Jiang Zemin, rule by *de* (roughly, virtue), but also correlates with the current political project of constructing a harmonious society, which is originally derived from Confucius's notion of *datong* (the Grand Union).

Masters of *guo xue* (national studies), such as Fu Peilong from Taiwan (2007a, 2007b), Yu Dan from Beijing Normal University (see Y. Zhang 2014 on Yu Dan's 2006 interpretation of the *Analects*), and Liu Yuli from the Central Party School of the Chinese Communist Party (Liu 2008), have delivered public lectures on how to use doctrines and precepts from Confucius and Mencius for psychological readjustment. These television lectures and teachings are then published as books or filmed as DVD. They discuss the basic principles and doctrines of Confucianism and their continued relevance and value in contemporary China. They contrast Confucian values, which are based on *ren* or *ren'ai* (compassion or love), with "Western" values, based on competition and "survival of the fittest." Then they explain the psychological mechanisms that cause mental and social imbalance in Chinese society. They discuss negative emotions, including anger, unhappiness, depression, stress, and envy, and common difficulties we encounter in a market economy, such as lack of trust, setbacks, competition, and betrayal, and the psychological adjustments they entail. The underlying messages include that one's psychological distress is not about difficulty or suffering, but the way we perceive and respond to such suffering; and that a moral person or a person with *de* (virtues) or *ren* (compassion) will not "encounter" such difficulties in the first place. In general, ancient stories, by historicizing certain values or ideologies, tend to intrigue audiences.

### Ren, Dao, *and moralizing psychology*

Confucius defines *ren* as love or compassion, "It is to love all men" (*Analects* 12:22). *Ren* is the value that one achieves in loving others. But he does not think loving others automatically results in *ren*. When asked by Yan Hui about *ren*, Confucius says it is "to subdue one's self and return to *li* [propriety]" (*Analects* 12:1). So *ren* is constrained by *li*. Moreover, he explains the notion of *ren* to Zhong Gong and Zi Gong by saying, "You yourself desire rank and standing; then help others to get rank and standing. You want to turn your own merits to account and then help turn theirs to account" (*Analects* 6:28). Thus, *ren* is actually the value that one achieves in the process of extending love from oneself to others. Throughout his life, Confucius set his heart upon the *Dao*, or the way of the social and natural order of the universe. Confucius said, "The *daos* of the true gentleman are threefold. I myself have met with success in none of them. For he who is really *ren* is never unhappy; he who is really wise is never perplexed; and he who is really brave is never afraid" (*Analects* 13:30). He can be seen as being modest here. However, these words do indicate that although a person who pursues *ren* can and should have no anxiety, this is not easy to achieve.

Liu Yuli (2008) points out that in the Western value system based on a capitalist market, self-centered, self-interested individuals are cultivated and competition is the norm, which leads to struggle and ultimately war. The fittest survives. In Confucian ethics, the self is based on relationships with others through mutual love and assistance. Ultimately, a world of *datong* (social harmony) is achieved. According to Liu, the Confucian notion of *wulun*, or five relationships (father–son, superior–subordinate, husband–wife, brother–brother, and friend–friend), which dominates Chinese society, is based on *ren* (compassion), not competition. The *Analects* discuss competition only once, and then the subject is shooting: *Junzi wu suo zheng, bu ye she hu; ti rang er sheng, xiang er yin, qi zheng ye junzi* – there is no competition for superior men; the only chance for them to compete is shooting, but even then, the process is based on humility and modesty. After they compete, they can still drink together. The winner will take the initiative to cheer up the loser with modesty and respect. Such competition is friendly, occurring between *junzi* (superior men). The loser does not resent the victor, but instead reflects on his own shortcoming or weakness. Here competition is not viewed as vicious and selfish acts, but is based on compassionate, ethical practices, which will inevitably gain those who practice *ren* more sustainable wealth and success.

Liu illustrates this point with the example of Chinese billionaire Li Jiacheng. During the 1973 oil crisis, the price of oil rose eightfold over pre-crisis prices. Instead of taking advantage of the crisis to gain profits, however, Li sold 20 tons of oil that he had in reserve to business owners – at half-price. He also organized other people who relied on oil for their businesses, so they could order oil in bulk from overseas, which lowered the purchase price. These benevolent acts saved many businesses in his industry, and those business owners regarded Li as their savior. Reciprocally, Li's *ren* gained him high respect and much assistance throughout the rest of his career, contributing to his current status and wealth.

As a counter-example of how *ren* facilitates health, happiness, and success, Liu tells the story of an official of the Song dynasty, named Jiang Yuan, who had nine sons, all of whom had physical disabilities except one, who died in prison. Another official, Gongming Zigao, asked Jiang about the possible reason for such misfortunes. Jiang told him that he was a jealous person. "Whenever I saw other people do good," he said, "I suspected their motivations; whenever I saw other people lose something, I felt like gaining something and was ecstatic; whenever I saw other people gain something, I resented them and felt like I lost something." Gongming persuaded Jiang to change his attitude and heart. After several years, all of Jiang Yuan's sons recovered. For Liu, envy of the kind Jiang had felt is destructive. It is derived from competition. *Ren*, meanwhile, gives rise to mutual assistance and mutual benefits – a win-win situation.

If we relate these parables to the values that are promoted through contemporary self-help in China, we can see that today's (new)Confucian ethics humanize market competition and enable people to cope with change, which implicitly serves government interests. This complementarity involves a particularly challenging paradox, as the goal is for people to forsake their individualistic orientations and root themselves in *ren*, while the government is moving in the opposite direction by creating a market economy that inevitably nurtures competition and individualism. Third force psychology, with its cooperative spirit of Confucianism, opens people's inner lives to participation in the developing market economy. This genre of ethical practice makes acceptance and openness to the fluctuations of the market into a kind of virtuous power to maintain equanimity in the face of change, while constraining one's ability or will to oppose government policy.

## CONCLUSION

One of Yu Dan's famous remarks, "Even if you have nothing to eat, your faith can also make you strong," might help summarize what *xinling jitang* is and how it may contribute to the political economy. Her remark is not that different from the kind of spiritual victory embedded in a popular *jitang* saying about smog in China: that it is the best defense against possible attacks from American laser weapons. But many Internet commentators stress that, regarding smog, we need more people like Li Guixin, who sued the director of the Shijiazhuang Bureau of Environmental Preservation on February 20, 2014, for the continuous air pollution in the city, rather than buying into *jitang*. Such messages embedded in *xinling jitang* often ignore social reality, neglect scientific facts, and are devoid of a social conscience. They are not that different from the slogans during Mao's era, "The output of the field depends on one's guts," or "Chairman Mao's thoughts can cure psychiatric diseases."

China's twin processes of privatization and marketization, including the reduction of medical and social services, have increasingly led individuals to make their own decisions. In stark contrast to life in the pre-reform era, when people tended to look up to the authority of the state for direction and guidance (see Chapter 6), individuals now are encouraged to become "experts" on their own, and learn to make their own choices, be responsible for themselves, and "help themselves." *Xinling jitang* in China, by turning inward and tapping into one's heart as a source of productivity and potentiality, not only mobilizes the masses to produce and compete in the market economy, but is also welcomed by the government to sustain sociopolitical stability. While in general *xinling jitang* promotes healing, happiness, and success, the overemphasis on the self, the inward turn, and positive consequences, which form a stark contrast with social reality, has backfired and attracted criticisms in China.

Instead of flattening psychology through the medical model of counseling in terms of health and illness, psychological training emphasizes the affective and performative force of psychology as a dynamic, pragmatic daily process. The emphasis on everyday life as a treasury for providing tools and technologies for psychological training shows a trend of psychologization that is more hegemonic and banal than the therapeutic governing of those who suffer from severe psychiatric disorders. Psychological self-help training as an ethical practice constructs a moral subject who fits a society based on Confucian ethics or the family-oriented political order. However, the popularization and vulgarization of Confucianism ultimately masks people's questioning of social reality and the meaning of life, offering only (politically) "correct" answers.

The recent turn to happiness in China is a turn toward psychology and affective life. Promoting happiness as therapy and as a mode of self-management is a way of governing socioeconomic issues in psychological terms. Much like communism or socialism, happiness points to a hope and a promise, creating a personal and political horizon that allows people to envision a good life (Ahmed 2010). However, the real control that occurs through happiness promotions or therapeutic governance is often unconscious; they optimize the individual's pleasurable fantasies and tie them to political and economic objectives. By turning economic stratification into the personal, emotional, and psychological and by optimizing happiness to incite pleasurable responses within subjects, thus minimizing opposition, such happiness promotions stabilize society.

The happiness industry in China, through (the rhetoric of) caring for people's well-being, appropriates happiness as an affect to intensify people's attachments to commodities, to certain incarnations of one another, and to the world. This process enhances consumerism and entrepreneurship. For a single-party state facing challenges in stabilizing society while integrating itself into the fast track of the global economy, the promotion of happiness for releasing positive and pre-empting negative potentials enhances social harmony and advances market development through such means as encouraging entrepreneurship and compliance among precariously employed workers.

The modes of self-realization in official happiness promotions are designed to endow individuals with new competencies and qualities. They are intended to make people feel better by enhancing their self-confidence and bringing them immediate relief from hardship. By orienting people away from social reality and toward their inner selves, and by constructing subjects who are psychologically obsessive but politically detached, this process appears to depoliticize social struggle and inequalities. However, the individualizing and psychologizing processes of happiness promotions and self-help also constitute new sites of contestation, as members of marginalized groups can take advantage of the government's advocacy of happiness and organize themselves in the name of enjoyment and happiness to protest collectively for their own benefits, as the laid-off workers in Changping did. The government's focus on the self will likely backfire for the state, as it will release a vast number of motivated individuals into society who are not satisfied with the offerings of the Party.

In general, the government not only uses psychology to provide a language or framework for people to interpret socioeconomic dislocation, but also integrates psychological forces into cultural and socioeconomic processes. Such psychologization apparently satisfies the contingent needs, interests, and aspirations of a certain class (i.e., entrepreneurs, psychotherapists, the state). Meanwhile, members of the working class and other underprivileged groups keep challenging this trend. The contestations occur even as China continues to promote happiness as the measure of a good life; such a parallel demonstrates that happiness has become both a nexus for contending with sociopolitical change and a tool for social critique.

# Conclusion: Psychologization and Therapeutic Governance

> When internal examination discovers nothing wrong, what is there to be
> anxious about, what is there to fear?
>
> Analects 3.12
>
> "A harmonious society" starts from the heart.
>
> *Liu Yuli 2008*

The most prominent emotional experience in China today is anxiety: political anxiety, economic anxiety, anxiety over belief, and anxiety over the future. Anxiety is China's (new) "epidemic." The remedy of choice is psychology, which makes sense to both the government and the people. In general, psychology's emphasis on the self and the inner life benefits the government: it distracts attention from government culpability for creating mental distress in the first place (through economic restructuring), makes individuals responsible for themselves (as opposed to the state), and advances market development (especially through the mental health industry). For the people, psychology, especially delivered in various self-help genres, offers accessible, non-stigmatizing treatment for distress with the veneer of moral direction.

Daniel Bell (2015) points to evidence of a political meritocracy at the top of China's political order, experimentation in the middle, and democracy at the bottom. One of the key issues Bell identifies in political meritocracy in China is the difficulty to legitimize the system to those outside the power structure. The problem of legitimacy can be addressed only by means of more opportunities for political participation, including some form of explicit consent by the people. He points out that Confucianism is one way to shape and justify China's political meritocracy. I would contend that, in a period of relentless change that began in the mid-1990s, psychology has become the conduit toward political meritocracy, enabling the Chinese government to directly engage the masses with psychological "care" and access their subjectivities through permissive empathy or by tapping into the popular psychological imagination to solicit the public's consent in managing certain social issues. For example, in the discourse of "officials' heartache," the government and media bank on the popular imagination of depression as biomedical, a move that downplays the sociopolitical forces that may contribute to Chinese officials' depression and suicide and constructs a façade of social harmony. If there is a problem, it is less with the legitimacy of psychology as a conduit for care amidst change, and more with the limits of psychology's capacity to address distress and reduce inequality imposed by its synthesis with governance. Indeed, the flexibility and adaptability of psychology have rendered it a subtle and powerful political technology that can transform issues requiring complex sociopolitical resolution into personal issues or pathology requiring "scientific" cures, but this process of psychologization – reduction, homogenization, or depoliticization – creates new vulnerabilities (especially for marginalized groups) and intensifies class stratification.

To my knowledge, this book is the first full-length study that combines theoretical concerns about the use of psychology by the Chinese state – that is, "therapeutic governance" – with attention to both psychiatry and psychosocial practices, particularly as they affect the construction of happiness, well-being, and gender in China. My ethnographic data address the impact of psychology's proliferation on a broad range of Chinese people, including members of China's elite, the middle class (i.e., Chinese officials), and underprivileged groups (i.e., laid-off workers). The book covers multiple interrelated factors

associated with mental illness in China: social, cultural, political, economic, and environmental. The mental health treatment models
include psychopharmaceutical-based hospital care, psychological counseling (online or face-to-face), genres of hybridizing counseling or psychological training with Chinese cultural traditions (Confucianism,
Daoism and Buddhism) and of blending counseling and nature-based
ecopsychology, and folk or faith healing. The focus of my analysis is
how these various mental health practices parallel, identify with, or are
co-opted by the government's interests and agendas, and how psychology, governance, political economy, and subjectivity inflect and fold into
one another, a process involving a concatenation of multiple powers:
disciplinary, biopolitical, necropolitical, stigmatic, and therapeutic. To
conclude the book, I summarize some of the key features of this
Chinese therapeutic governance by considering both culture and
phenomenology.

First, it is a turn based in history. The work units that once served
as the basic organizing mechanism for Chinese society since Mao's time
have been gradually dismantled as a result of China's economic restructuring. These units were a medium between the people and the government, the basis of providing urbanites with material, emotional, and
spiritual support, and a safety valve that could absorb social complaints
and resolve social conflicts. With the gradual collapse of work units,
the government has been compelled to find alternative mechanisms to
reconnect to the people. Psychology and therapeutic governance are
such means. Through psychologization of social issues and permissive
empathy embedded in the relationship between the state/therapist and
the people/client, the government reaches the hearts and minds of
individuals. While "caring" for the people and emphasizing their private
and inner lives, the government also turns their attention away from
broader socioeconomic processes, thereby seeking to avert social criticism and possible collective unrest, promoting stability. That is, the
government cares only insofar as caring allows it to govern. In general,

psychologization skews a (psycho)therapeutic ethos to legitimate and facilitate the current socialist project of building the harmonious society. The theme of the 2016 World Mental Health Day in China, for example, was *xinli jiankang, hexie shehui* (Psychological Health, Harmonizing Society) – a synthesis of mental health and sociopolitical stability.

This historical genealogy can be seen, for example, in the lingering impact of the traditional Communist ideological orientation – thought work – on psychotherapy, which has made CBT one of the most prominent types of counseling in China. Its pragmatic and directive features and its focus on remaking one's thoughts through practical measures echo thought work. In other words, thought work finds a new incarnation in psychological counseling. Social and political differences and "deviances" are now more pathologized than politicized.

In this historical genealogy, we can also see therapeutic governance taking place in the context of the moral and psychological "vacuum" created by a decline in the acceptance of Communist ideology by ordinary people, a growing lack of social support, and the absence of a new social and moral ideology beyond market economics. Instead of revising its political vision and economic policies in ways that would soften the negative impact of rapid socioeconomic change, government programs promoting happiness and psychotherapy seek to compel individuals to become responsible for their own care in order to harness their positive potentials for sociopolitical stabilization and economic development. This mode of therapeutic governance constitutes a channel for the state to re-engage the masses in order to regain their recognition and trust amidst economic restructuring after losing the mediation of the work unit system.[1] This "caring" form of governing apparently renews the Party's "socialist" commitment. Psychology has thus become a tool for building idealistic situations that parallel or identify with longstanding "socialist" ideals (i.e., the common refrain of social harmony).

Second, therapeutic governance in China embraces informal diagnosis. It does not entirely rely on the expertise of medical authority. Government agencies, institutions, and even individuals can "diagnose" people as suffering from certain mental illness and put them in mental health facilities. Such informal diagnosis can also be applied to dead bodies, for example in the case of officials' suicides. This necropolitics and the dispensability of medical expertise in mental illness diagnosis not only de-professionalize medicine, but also highlight the capricious and sovereign aspect of this governance. In this sense, psy experts occupy an ambivalent position between the state and the masses in China in recent years when experts and expertise have increasingly shaped politics.

The practice of informal diagnosis may partly derive from the tradition of mass mobilization during Mao's era: people were mobilized to spy on one another as "thought police," assigned to assess one another's ideological conformity with Chairman Mao's thoughts. Now, instead of political "correctness," the masses tend to use psychological discourse and therapeutic terms to scrutinize and diagnose family members, neighbors, and those around them for mental disorders. In general, informal diagnoses capitalize on and reinforce the psychological knowledge that has become part of the popular imagination, including stigma associated with mental disorders. This gives rise to overpsychologization and overdiagnosis, highlighting the growing cultural authority of psychology in Chinese society.

Third, therapeutic governance is supported by stigma. Stigma associated with mental disorders in China attaches not only to the individual who suffers from mental distress, but also to his or her family and community. It is an informal mode of control and governing. In the context of China's emphasis on *minben* (i.e., the government's moral orientation toward benefiting the people), stigma also constitutes a site of contestation and even a way for those who suffer mental disorders and their families to allocate resources. Persistent stigma surrounding mental illness has partly facilitated China's psychoboom, especially the mushrooming self-help genres, through which people familiarize themselves with knowledge of mental illness and attempt to heal themselves without risking loss of "face." While the state has endorsed efforts to destigmatize mental illness, these efforts tend to promote a biomedical view of mental illness, which ultimately supports a status quo of biomedicine and economic growth. Celebrities like Cui Yongyuan can now reveal their personal experiences with depression treatment. This destigmatizes depression. But it also highlights the condition as a highly individualized pathology, which tends to foreclose the possibility of socially induced depression – situational depression. In this sense, stigma attached to mental illness legitimates the predominantly biomedical treatment in Chinese mental hospitals and boosts the psychopharmaceutical industry, while sidelining talk therapy or socioeconomic conditions leading to distress.

Fourth, therapeutic governance intensifies gender and class inequalities. It prioritizes some groups over others and optimizes resources for the interests of elite and managerial classes and the government. Inevitably, this intensifies inequalities between classes, and between men and women. For example, while with state enterprise restructuring and mass layoffs, members of the working class have been reportedly more prone to anger, depression, and suicide than have other classes, psychiatric and psychotherapeutic resources are more accessible to members of urban middle and elite classes. Essentialized psychological discourse tends to target women and their psychological states, but does so in ways that uphold men as the standard of humanity. In various forms of care, ideal female subjects are constructed as happy, well-adjusted "wise mothers" and "virtuous wives" for the home and family, all of which serves the interest of men and the state. This essentialized role of women can take the place of state social support, as women are encouraged to fulfill their destiny as caregivers. Meanwhile, both gender and mental distress, which have been constructed more biologically in the official discourses than in Mao's era, can be mobilized to express (class) differences, downplaying social stratifications and inequalities intensified by privatization.

Fifth, therapeutic governance accesses the heart. Chinese psychological practices, by invoking the heart as a moral core of subjectivity, a venue for knowledge production, and a fundamental component of being, render such practices more attuned to subjective experiences and personal feelings, endow therapeutic governance with greater efficacy in reaching Chinese hearts and minds, and realize more thorough internal transcendence (*neizai chaoyue*) than typically psyche-based Western psychology. The heart thus distinguishes *xinli hua* from typical Western pscyhologization. Rendering social and cultural practices through the lens of the heart, *xinli hua* not only psychologizes, but also looks at the "heart" – or true nature – of these practices. In this sense, unlike the reductive process of psychologization, *xinli hua* involves intensification and depth in its rendering. Meanwhile, pointing to the outside, knowledge of the heart, in recent conceptualizations by Chinese counselors, tends to attach to intersubjective dimensions of experience rather than broader social processes. The focus on interiority or the heart does not downplay the impact of the self and its dialogic interaction with the external world in the Chinese context. Rather, this internalizing process guides people to question their own heart-attitude or mental capacities rather than look at social conditions when faced with a crisis. These paradoxical characteristics of the Chinese heart make therapeutic practices and governing ambiguous, porous, and hegemonic.

Sixth, therapeutic governance enhances commercialization. China's economic restructuring has led to a reduction in government health insurance. Responsibility for funding public health care has shifted dramatically from the central state to local authorities and hospitals, which are profit-driven. This, in turn, makes mental health services more expensive and less accessible to most Chinese. Concurrently, the country has experienced a psychoboom. I argue that these phenomena – retrenchment of social support and proliferation of psychology – are connected and show some degree of complicity between the state and market. Big pharmaceutical companies and the state devise strategies to mask their influence in this shift and promote the idea that feelings and opinions of individuals originate solely from within the individual. This (neoliberal) model of society and psychological discourse stresses that individuals take responsibility for the deficiencies and injustice they experience. Meanwhile, psychology provides a new terrain for enhancement and productivity: the realm of interiority, including the heart, emotion, subconsciousness, and potentiality. For example, the kind of emotion management (i.e., happiness) promoted through psychologization cultivates an entrepreneurial, therapeutic subject who is self-caring, self-motivated, and self-sufficient and who can accomplish anything. Further, the predominance of biomedicine in Chinese mental hospitals boosts the development of psychopharmacology and the mental health industry.

Seventh, therapeutic governance deploys tradition as a resource. Since the 1990s, the Chinese government has selectively promoted cultural tradition as part of its political values.[2] Since then, its ongoing promotion has kept pace with a weakening of ideological control over the people. For example, given that Confucianism stands for order, hierarchy, and tradition, its revitalization assists with government attempts to regain authority. More generally, the revitalization of Buddhism, Daoism, and Confucianism has been used to promote and further the reach of psychologization and therapeutic governance. The emphasis on cultural tradition as a resource for psychological relief demonstrates how psychology, morality, tradition, and politics are integrated into an emerging psychopolitical economy in China. Chinese psychologists and Confucian philosophers moralize, psychologize, and repoliticize elements of this tradition, with an emphasis on the heart as the moral core of individual agency to achieve equanimity to cope with anxiety and stress. To some extent, the heart acts as the linchpin combining the psychological, the moral, and the political.

The revitalization of these traditional cultural resources to meet contemporary needs and alleviate the pressure of China's modernization serves to deepen the government's reach of the heart-minds of individuals and add depth, credibility, and legitimacy to Chinese psy experts' adoption of Western psychology. As I point out in Chapter 6, however, "re-traditionalization" has not uniformly turned attention away from situational causes of distress. Many Chinese psy professionals do see the effects of socioeconomic dislocation. These professionals endeavor to address psychological pain through a combination of cognitive-based psychological treatment with affect-based approaches, for example by drawing on culturally sensitive healing resources. However, many more, in part owing to an overburdened system that leaves them with few resources to address deeper causes, tend to offer "pragmatic," cost-efficient treatment, mostly through variations of CBT, pharmaceuticals, and even electroconvulsive therapy. Such biomedical or cognitive approaches to mental health might be part of the problem, contributing to the large-scale mental health "crisis."

In sum, by addressing phenomenology and social and cultural specificity in China, this analysis of therapeutic governance shows that mental distress is not only about psychological responses to social, economic, and political transformations but also about culturally mediated experiences with power and injustice. Today's Chinese state is not entirely cold-hearted. As represented by mental health practitioners who have been trained in officially funded institutions, the government does make genuine attempts to alleviate distress. But given the scope of anxiety and mental distress in China, state mental health interventions are more tokens of care and benevolence than solutions and a source of real relief. This hints that care is not an end in itself. My argument is that the state needs psychology as a kind of prop: psychology masks the inadequacy of other social and governing resources. It obscures the possibility of more complex, responsible approaches to socioeconomic issues. Indeed, psychologization of social and political issues cannot replace laws for governing or the reform of structural forces that generate distress. Using psychology, the state can problematize and reshape events and activities, difficulties and distress into phenomena requiring expert intervention and individual efforts.

As a "positive" and "soft" mode of intervention, psychology is seen by the current government as a feasible model for reforming those who are not well adjusted to change and who are distressed. Ultimately, psychology has become part of a new language that speaks to people about rebuilding their identities around an emotional core that obfuscates the socioeconomic dislocation they experience. Psychologization contributes to and profits from the general trend in the 1990s that delegitimized the moral and political judgments about sociopolitical deviances and replaced them with "scientific facts." It helps the state and the people remake themselves in preparation for a future in which yet more competition and economic growth are expected. With the government assistance and the veneer of tradition in psychologization, the new Chinese subject is expected to be moral, independent, and willing to work on personal failings.

# Notes

Introduction: China's Mental Health "Crisis"?

1 As of the 1990s, well over 90 percent of the 4.8 million persons with schizophrenia in China lived with family members (Phillips 1993).

2 Falun Gong, a traditional form of *qigong*, is rooted in ancient Chinese culture. The practice won the hearts of many by adhering to spiritual principles independent of the state (Lu and Galli 2002). Falun Gong can bring health and psychiatric benefits, and was once lauded for saving the government tremendous resources. Persecution of practitioners reportedly stemmed from its popularity: by 1997 its 70 million adherents far exceeded Chinese Communist Party membership (about 50 million) (Lu and Galli 2002).

3 This echoes what Sing Lee (1998) calls "traveling psychosis" among rural migrants, a contested diagnosis concerning a severe mental disturbance that occurs among migrant workers who travel long distance in China's overcrowded trains.

4 In 2009, China's Ministry of Science invested 40 million yuan (US$16 million) in research projects, including suicide prevention and reducing occupational stress (Chen 2010). International NGOs and donors have also been involved in promoting community-based psychological relief initiatives.

5 The Confucian self, with its emphasis on collective ambiance and the heart, is more disposed toward self-reflexivity and self-governing than is the autonomous self.

6 Such informal diagnostic procedures can be applied in appointing Chinese officials. Shao Jingjun (2016), a specialist researcher at the Central Disciplinary Committee of the Chinese Communist Party, defines jealousy, violence, revenge, stubbornness, self-aggrandizement, narcissism, dependence, indifference, flattery, and habitual lying as psychological illnesses that partly contribute to rampant corruption among Chinese officials without appealing to medical expertise.

7   Bed-warming services are mainly performed by women, who will warm the bed, run baths, and so on, mainly for white-collar workers before they return home from work in China's big cities.

8   "Loneliness Nurtures Companion Economy." WeChat: *Nanfang Ribao*, February 16, 2017 (in Chinese).

9   I translated all Chinese texts and interview data.

**Chapter 1   Mental Health and Mental Illness: Concepts and Contradictions**

1   http://mp.weixin.qq.com/s?__biz=MjM5MDk1MDE4MQ==&mid=2650777690&idx=1&sn=22018010b02186ccfd43c91c3192ee29&scene=0#wechat_redirect.

2   Zhou (2014) contends that in a sense, the sources of today's social anxiety can be dated back to the 1840s, when China was defeated in the Opium War (1839–42) by the Western powers and forced to open its doors.

3   China's suicide rate is around 23 per 100,000 people, far exceeding the world average of 13 per 100,000 people (Liu 2016).

4   According to government figures, between August 2003 and April 2014, 112 officials committed suicide in China. This number is misleading because most suicides among officials are not reported. For example, only four officials reportedly committed suicide in 2013. Yet during the first half of 2013, 6,526 out of 10 million public servants in China went missing: 8,371 escaped overseas, and 1,252 took their lives (Qi 2013).

5   This phenomenon defies the general situation that in China women are on average more depressive than men (Qin et al. 2015).

6   As *guo lao si* (overwork death) in China is blamed on one's original physical and psychological illnesses exacerbated by overwork, officials' suicides are attributed to their psychological (and physical) fragility.

7   http://pinglun.eastday.com/p/20110714/u1a5995236.html.

**Chapter 2   New Chinese Mental "Illnesses"**

1   Research on *xinfang* as a governmental practice to funnel people's grievances and complaints often focuses on the strategic logic or the rights consciousness of petitioners, the organizational tactics of protestors, and the costs undertaken by local government to suppress cases and structural differentiation within the state (Perry 2002; Cai 2004; Deng and O'Brien 2013).

2   Before 1997, suicide in this community was rare and primarily confined to women.

3 "China Now World's Largest Online Gaming Market." CGTN, January 8, 2016 (https://america.cgtn.com/2016/01/08/china-now-worlds-largest-online-gaming-market).

4 "Cure Your Children's Internet Addiction with Electric Shocks Aversion Therapy." China Hush, May 14, 2009 (http://www.chinahush.com/2009/05/14/cure-your-childrens-internet-addiction-with-electric-shocks-aversion-therapy/).

5 On January 6, 2017, China's Department of Internet and Communication drafted new rules to regulate Internet use by youth, including a curfew on Internet surfing between midnight and 8:00 a.m., smartphones to be equipped with software protecting youth from Internet gaming, and a ban on coercive treatment of Internet addiction (Beijing Youth Daily, January 7, 2017).

6 Both the concept of kongxin bing and statistics are controversial: an article in the People's Daily considers kongxin bing part of students' growing pains rather than a psychological disorder (Chang 2016).

**Chapter 3 Gender, Class, and Mental Health**

1 One exception is migrant workers. Qin and colleagues (2015) studied the mental health status of migrant workers in Shanghai. They found that 25 percent of men and 6 percent of women suffer from various kinds of mental disorders. The sharp gender difference may be either because of the higher work-related stress men experience or because more men than women migrate to cities for jobs (see Lee 1998 on traveling psychosis).

2 "Professional Women Are More Depressed than Men." WeChat: Yiyuzheng, January 16, 2017 (in Chinese).

3 This discourse pathologizes four types of "poisonous" motherhood or mother–daughter relationships as full of negativity, anger, emotional control, and harm (Xiao Lou 2016), and condemns mothers who are contemptuous, controlling, cold and evasive, or encroaching on the boundary of self and offspring.

4 "What Are the Biggest Obstacles in Counseling for the Public?" The 2016 Psychological Counseling Industry Report. WeChat: Yi Xinli, July 20, 2016 (in Chinese).

5 The only blue-collar workers who presumably suffer symptoms of xiangpi ren are taxi-drivers because they are more targeted for counseling as they act as the "windows" (the public face) of cities (J. Yang 2015).

6 Interestingly, beauty criteria in China, while based on "Western" standards, are often filtered through Korean beauty products and cosmetics culture.

### Chapter 4 Stigma and Control

1 Goffman first introduces the concept of face and defines it as "an image of self delineated in terms of approved social attributes" (2005: 5).
2 "Postpartum Depression: New Mothers Are More Vulnerable Than You Imagine." WeChat: *Yiyuzheng*, August 8, 2016 (in Chinese).
3 "Depression Cannot be Cured by 'Thinking Out.'" WeChat: *Yiyuzheng*, August 10, 2016 (in Chinese).
4 "Depression is Not Your Fault." WeChat: *Yiyuzheng*, September 14, 2016 (in Chinese).

### Chapter 5 Psychopharmacology, Subjectivity, and Psychiatric Hospital Care

1 Psychiatry was founded in China with the establishment of the first psychiatric hospital by Western missionaries in Guangzhou, Guangdong Province, in 1898 (Chiang 2014). In Mao's era, mental illness was perceived as a vestige of bourgeois ideology. Psychiatry did not just cure the sick body with medication but also aimed to heal pathological sociality through ideological and social intervention. During the Cultural Revolution, psychiatry was misused to label and incarcerate political dissidents as mentally ill (Munro 2002).
2 "The Treatment of Depression through CBT" WeChat: *MedSci*, June 5, 2016 (in Chinese).

### Chapter 6 Counseling and Indigenous Psychology

1 To facilitate the growth of psychology in China, Fu Chunsheng (2016), director of Zhongke Bo'ao Psychological Hospital, suggests that five models be adopted: (1) counseling: both one-on-one face-to-face and online; (2) employee assistance programs (EAP), focusing on clients' real concerns and sources of pressure, which actually come more from employees' family duties than work; (3) psychological training, focusing on small-scale training sessions (i.e., salons or workshops); (4) organizing profit-making psychological conferences; and, finally, (5) developing new psychological products.
2 CTCP is an instructive treatment based on eight Daoist principles encompassed in 32 Chinese characters from the *Daodejing*: (1) 利而不害 (Benefit without harm to yourself and others); (2) 為而不爭

(Do your best without competition with others); (3) 少私寡慾 (Limit selfishness and moderate desire); (4) 知足知止 (Know when to stop and learn how to be satisfied); (5) 知和處下 (Know harmony and be humble); (6) 以柔制剛 (Hold softness to defeat hardness); (7) 返樸歸真 (Return to purity and innocence); and (8) 順其自然 (Follow the rule of nature). In clinical application, therapists explain to and guide patients as opposed to engaging in behaviors such as self-exploration (Zhang et al. 2002). A Daoist worldview is characterized by principles of acceptance, balance, and harmony with natural laws, and non-action (*wuwei*). These values have been used to relieve mental suffering since ancient China (Cheng et al. 2010).

3 China's psychoboom has allowed certain "gurus" to drive the development of hybrid counseling methods, partly because people like the idea of clarity and authority. They are predominantly male academics or medical practitioners, affiliated with public universities or hospitals. They are popular and wealthy published authors. Most of them are trained in both China and the West; their counseling is usually government-sponsored or -approved.

4 ICP also draws on Carl Jung's notion of active imagination, a form of guided imagery. Jung contends that an image can convey a meaning or symbolism far greater than we can describe in words. When one concentrates on a mental picture, it begins to stir; the image becomes enriched by details. Without interrupting the natural flow of events, one's unconscious will produces a series of images that makes a complete story (Jung 1961).

5 Gesang Zeren, Professor of Psychology at Sichuan University, created another Chinese psychotherapeutic practice called *dejue cuimian* (*dejue* hypnosis), which combines elements of Tibetan Buddhism, Tibetan medicine, and Chinese wisdom of life-nurturing with Western hypnotic techniques. *Dejue* advocates the communication between two selves: the true self, revealing one's true character, and the other, a mask to hide one's real personality, in order to achieve a perfect balance – relaxation and freedom from the lure of wealth and power.

6 Wu (2016) argues that *juying* is at *kou yu qi* (the oral stage), according to Freud's five psychosexual developmental stages.

7 The philosophy is captured in Zheng's passage: "*Congming nan, hutu nan, you congming er zhuanru hutu geng nan. Fang yizhao, tui yibu, dang xia xin an, fei tu houlai fu bao ye* [Being bright is not easy. But it's also difficult being muddled. If you start out being bright, it is even harder to be muddled. Let go! Step back! If you want to have present peace

of mind, don't anticipate future rewards]" (Matthyssen 2012; see also Matthyssen 2015).

8 EMDR uses bilateral stimulation or eye movement to activate the opposite sides of the brain, releasing emotional experiences that are "trapped" in the nervous system (Shapiro and Laliotis 2010).

### Chapter 7  Happiness and Psychological Self-Help

1 "Why Does Self-Help Literature Not Benefit You?" WeChat: *Linzi Xinlitang*, August 30, 2016 (in Chinese).

2 Yu Dan, Professor of Media Studies at Beijing Normal University, became famous for lecturing on Confucianism at CCTV's Lecture Room.

3 Lei Feng, a soldier of the People's Liberation Army, was well known for his selfless behavior in performing his duty and wholeheartedly helping others. After he died on duty in 1962, Chairman Mao designated him a martyr for the revolutionary cause (see J. Yang 2015).

### Conclusion:  Psychologization and Therapeutic Governance

1 This can be reflected in the shift of channels of Chinese people's petitioning. A 2015 survey (Zhang 2016) shows that if encountering social injustice, 71.3 percent of the people choose to go to court and 15.9 percent go to petition through the *xinfang* system, while only 13.8 percent return to their work units for a resolution (compared to 72 percent in 1987). In 2013, less than one quarter of the urban population still remained in the typical work unit system.

2 China established its *guoxue zhongxin* (Center for National Studies) in Beijing in October 2016. The government has decided to promote classic national studies in China's elementary and middle school system. "China's National Studies Center Was Complete." WeChat: *Rujiawang Zongheshijian*, October 8, 2016 (in Chinese).

# References

A Su. 2014. "Money Hunger Disease is a Social Epidemic." WeChat: *Tongdao Xinling Gongzuoshi*, November 14 (in Chinese).

Ahmed, Sara. 2004. *The Cultural Politics of Emotion*. New York: Routledge.

Ahmed, Sara. 2010. *The Promise of Happiness*. Durham, NC: Duke University Press.

Bartlett, Nicholas. 2016. "Idling in Mao's Shadow: Heroin Addiction and the Contested Therapeutic Value of Socialist Traditions of Laboring." *Culture, Medicine and Psychiatry*. doi:10.1007/s11013-016-9512-9.

Bateson, Gregory. 1973. *Steps to an Ecology of Mind*. New York: Paladin.

Bax, Trent. 2014. *Youth and Internet Addiction in China*. Abingdon: Routledge.

Bedford, Olwen and Kwang-Kuo Hwang. 2003. "Guilt and Shame in Chinese Culture: A Cross-cultural Framework from the Perspective of Morality and Identity." *Journal for the Theory of Social Behavior* 33 (2): 127–44.

Bell, Daniel A. 2008. *China's New Confucianism: Politics and Everyday Life in a Changing Society*. Princeton: Princeton University Press.

Bell, Daniel A. 2015. *The Chinese Model: Political Meritocracy*. Princeton: Princeton University Press.

Bi Shumin. 2008. *Xinli Zixun Shouji* [Notes on Psychological Counseling]. Beijing: China Youth Press.

Bi Shumin. 2012. *Mei you ren shi yi zuo gudao* [No Man is an Island]. Changsha, Hunan Province: Hunan Wenyi Chubanshe.

Biehl, João, Byron J. Good, and Arthur Kleinman. 2007. "Introduction: Rethinking Subjectivity." In *Subjectivity: Ethnographic Investigations*, eds. João Biehl, Byron J. Good, and Arthur Kleinman. Berkeley: University of California Press.

Björkell, Stina. 2011. "Eating Disorders in China: A Sign of the Times." *GB Times*, February 15. http://gbtimes.com/life/eating-disorders-china-sign-times.

Blume, Lawrence. 2002. "Stigma and Social Control." Institute for Advanced Studies, Vienna. http://www.ssc.wisc.edu/econ/Durlauf/networkweb1/wpapers/es-119.pdf.

Bond, Michael H. 1986. "Mutual Stereotypes and the Facilitation of Interaction across Cultural Lines." *International Journal of Intercultural Relations* 10: 259–76.

Borovoy, Amy. 2005. *The Too-Good Wife: Alcohol, Codependency, and the Politics of Nurturance in Postwar Japan.* Berkeley: University of California Press.

Brady, Anne-Marie. 2008. *Marketing Dictatorship: Propaganda and Thought Work in Contemporary China.* Lanham, MD: Rowman & Littlefield Publishers.

Brownell, Susan. 1995. *Training the Body for China: Sports in the Moral Order of the People's Republic.* Chicago: University of Chicago Press.

Bunkenborg, Mikkel. 2014. "Subhealth: Questioning the Quality of Bodies in Contemporary China." *Medical Anthropology* 33: 128–43.

Busfield, Joan. 1989. *Managing Madness: Changing Ideas and Practices.* London: Unwin Hyman Ltd.

Busfield, Joan. 2012. "Gender and Mental Health." In *The Palgrave Handbook of Gender and Healthcare,* eds. Ellen Kuhlmann and Ellen Annadale. London: Macmillan.

Busfield, Joan. 2014. "Gender and Mental Illness." In *The Wiley Blackwell Encyclopedia of Health, Illness, Behavior, and Society,* eds. William C. Cockerham, Robert Dingwall, and Stella R. Quah. London: Wiley-Blackwell.

Cai, Yongshun. 2004. "Managed Participation in China." *Political Science Quarterly* 119 (3): 425–51.

Chang Yu. 2016. "Empty Heart Disease May Be a False Claim." *People's Daily,* November 19 (in Chinese).

Chen Anzhi. 2016. "Whether a Child is Outstanding or Not is Determined by Her Mother's Personality." WeChat: *Chen Anzhi,* August 28 (in Chinese).

Chen, Feng. 1994. "The Dilemma of Eudaemonic Legitimacy in Post-Mao China." *Polity* XXIX (3): 422–35.

Chen, Nancy N. 2003. *Breathing Spaces: Qi, Psychiatry and Healing in China.* New York: Columbia University Press.

Chen, Xi. 2014. *Social Protest and Contentious Authoritarianism in China.* Cambridge: Cambridge University Press.

Chen Zewei. 2010. "Resolving the Pain/Threats Posed by the Mentally Ill." *Outlook Weekly,* May 31 (in Chinese).

Cheng, Cecilia, Barbara C.Y. Lo, and Jasmine H.M. Chio. 2010. "The Tao (Way) of Chinese Coping." In *The Oxford Handbook of Chinese Psychology,* ed. Michael H. Bond. New York: Oxford University Press.

Chesler, Phyllis. 1972. *Women and Madness.* Ann Arbor: University of Michigan Press.

Chiang, Howard (Ed.). 2014. *Psychiatry and Chinese History.* London: Pickering & Chatto.

Chu Zhaoxian. 2011. "Official Fear: Inside a *Shuanggui* Investigation Facility". *Dui Hua: Human Rights Journal,* July 5. http://www.duihuahrjournal.org/2011/07/official-fear-inside-shuanggui.html.

Clay, Rebecca A. 2002. "Chinese Psychology." *Monitor on Psychology* 33 (3): 64.

Cloward, Richard A. and Frances F. Piven. 1979. "Hidden Protest: The Channeling of Female Innovation and Resistance." *Signs* 4 (4): 651–69.

Corrigan, Patrick W. and Amy C. Watson. 2002. "Understanding the Impact of Stigma on People with Mental Illness." *World Psychology* 1 (1): 16–20.

Cui, Jianping (*jia fei mao*). 2011. *Nihao, Xiao Que Xing* [Hello, Small but Certain Happiness]. Nanjing: Fenghuang Chubanshe.

Cushman, Philip. 1992. "Psychotherapy to 1992: A Historically Situated Interpretation." In *History of Psychotherapy: A Century of Change,* ed. Donald K. Freedheim. Washington, DC: American Psychological Association.

Deng, Yanhua and Kevin J. O'Brien. 2013. "Relational Repression in China: Using Social Ties to Demobilize Protesters." *The China Quarterly* 215: 533–52.

Dolby, Sandra K. 2005. *Self-Help Books: Why Americans Keep Reading Them.* Urbana and Chicago: University of Illinois Press.

Dong Bihui. 2014. "Obsession with Iron Rice Bowl is a Disease and Needs to Be Treated." *Qianjiang Evening Newspaper,* November 19 (in Chinese). http://star.news.sohu.com/20141119/n406162537.shtm.

Economist Intelligence Unit. 2016. "Mental Health and Integration – Provision for Supporting People with Mental Illness: A Comparison of 15 Asia Pacific Countries." https://www.eiuperspectives.economist.com/sites/default/files/Mental_health_and_integration.pdf.

Ehrenberg, Alain. 2010. *The Weariness of the Self: Diagnosing the History of Depression in the Contemporary Age.* Montreal: McGill-Queens University Press.

Ewen, Stewart. 1989. "Advertising and the Development of Consumer Society." In *Cultural Politics in Contemporary America,* eds. Ian Angus and Sut Jhally. New York: Routledge.

Fan Junjuan. 2016. "Chinese Men Are Critically 'Sick.'" WeChat: *Xingzhi Zueyuan,* January 29 (in Chinese).

Fang Kecheng, Yun Anqi, and Zhang Lu. 2011. "'Officials' Heartache': How Much Do You Know?" *South China Weekly,* December 8 (in Chinese).

Farquhar, Judith. 2001. "For Your Reading Pleasure: Popular Health Advice and the Anthropology of Everyday Life in 1990s Beijing." *Positions* 9 (1): 105–30.

Farquhar, Judith and Qicheng Zhang. 2012. *Ten Thousand Things: Nurturing Life in Contemporary Beijing.* New York: Zone Books.

Fei Xiaotong. 1999. "Zhongguo Chengxiang Fazhan de Daolu: Wo Yisheng de Yanjiu Keti [The Road of Chinese Rural–Urban Development: My Lifetime Topic]." In *Fei Xiaotong Wenji* [Collections of Fei Xiaotong's Works], Vol. 12. Beijing: Qunyan Publishing House.

Fei Xiaotong. 1992. *From the Soil: The Foundations of Chinese Society.* Berkeley: University of California Press.

Feng, Jicai. 1996. *Ten Years of Madness: Oral Histories of China's Cultural Revolution.* San Francisco: China Books.

Flam, Helena. 2004. "Anger in Repressive Regimes: A Footnote to Domination and the Arts of Resistance by James Scott." *European Journal of Social Theory* 7 (2): 171–88.

Foucault, Michel. 1976. *Mental Illness and Psychology.* New York: Harper & Row.

Foucault, Michel. 1978. *The History of Sexuality: An Introduction.* New York: Pantheon Books.

Foucault, Michel. 1998. *Aesthetics, Methods and Epistemology: Essential Works of Foucault, 1954–1984*, Vol. II, ed. James D. Faubion. New York: New Press.

Friedan, Betty. 1965. *The Feminine Mystique.* Harmondsworth: Penguin.

Friedman, Jack. 2016. "A World Crazier Than Us: Vanishing Social Contexts and the Consequences for Psychiatric Practice in Contemporary Romania." *Transcultural Psychiatry* 53 (2): 176–97.

Fu Chunsheng. 2016. "The Five Models for Psychological Institutes to Grow." WeChat: *Xinli Gongkaike*, July 24 (in Chinese).

Fu Peilong. 2007a. *Xiang Kongzi Wen Dao* [Learning Dao from Confucius]. Beijing: Chinese International Broadcasting Publisher.

Fu Peilong. 2007b. *Xiang Mengzi Wen Dao* [Learning Dao from Mencius]. Beijing: Chinese International Broadcasting Publisher.

Furedi, Frank. 2004. *Therapy Culture: Cultivating Vulnerability in an Uncertain Age.* London: Routledge.

Gao Chengxin and Liu Jie. 2016. "Always Feeling Depressed? Learning About Depression Through Three Dimensions." WeChat: *Shehuixue Le Mei (Isocialor)*, June 9 (in Chinese).

Gao Shiyuan and Michael R. Phillips. 2001. "Attitudes About Mental Illness of Different Types of Respondents in Beijing." *Chinese Mental Health* 15: 107–9.

Goffman, Erving. 2005. *Interaction Ritual: Essays in Face-to-Face Behavior.* New Brunswick, NJ: Transaction.

Goldstein, Robert L. 1987. "Litigious Paranoids and the Legal System: The Role of the Forensic Psychiatrist." *Journal of Forensic Sciences* 32 (4): 1009–15.

Good, Byron J. 1977. "The Heart of What's the Matter: The Semantics of Illness in Iran." *Culture, Medicine and Psychiatry* 1: 25–58.

Goodman, David. 2014. *Class in China*. Cambridge: Polity.

Gordon, Colin. 1991. "Governmental Rationality: An Introduction." In *The Foucault Effect: Studies in Governmentality*, eds. Graham Burchell, Colin Gordon, and Peter Miller. Chicago: University of Chicago Press.

Green, Michael F. 2003. *Schizophrenia Revealed: From Neurons to Social Interactions*. New York and London: Sage.

Gu Baoxing. 2013. "God Can Only Help You Find the Wound." WeChat: *Lingdao Wencui*, November 20 (in Chinese).

Gu, Jun, Chen-Bo Zhong, and Elizabeth Page-Gould. 2013. "Listen to Your Heart: When False Somatic Feedback Shapes Moral Behavior." *Journal of Experimental Psychology* 142 (2): 307–12.

Guo, Feng and Terry Hanley. 2015. "Adapting Cognitive Behavioral Therapy to Meet the Needs of Chinese Clients: Opportunities and Challenges." *PsyCh Journal* 4: 55–65.

Guo, Jinhua. 2016. *Stigma: An Ethnography of Mental Illness and HIV/AIDS in China*. Hackensack: World Century.

Hacking, Ian. 1986. "Making up People." In *Reconstructing Individualism: Autonomy, Individuality, and the Self in Western Thought*, eds. Thomas C. Heller, Morton Sosna, and David E. Wellbery. Stanford: Stanford University Press.

Hall, David L. and Roger T. Ames. 1998. *Thinking through the Han: Self, Truth and Transcendence in Chinese and Western Culture*. Albany, NY: State University of New York Press.

Han Buxin and Zhang Kan. 2007. "Psychology in China." *The Psychologist* 20: 734–6.

Han Haoyue. 2010. "Fake Happiness Diverts Disadvantaged Groups' Attention from Social Inequalities." March 18 (in Chinese). http://cul.sohu.com/20100318/n270928949.shtml.

Han Yan. 2016. "*Xinli Hua*: Understanding Others and the World from the Heart's Perspective." WeChat: *Shifen Xinli*, October 20 (in Chinese).

Hanser, Amy. 2008. *Service Encounters: Class, Gender, and the Market for Social Distinction in Urban China*. Stanford, CA: Stanford University Press.

Hao Wanshan. 2014. *Bu Shengqi Jiu Bu Shengbing* [No Anger, No Sickness]. Taiwan: Dongfang Chubanshe.

He Jun. 2016. "The Humanity Factor in Men's Depression." WeChat: *Jiuzhou Xinli*, June 9 (in Chinese).

He Qinglian. 2011. "Who Makes China a Big Country of Mental Sickness" (in Chinese). http://voachineseblog.com/heqinglian/2011/10/mental-sickness-china/.

Hill, Napoleon. 1937/1953. *Think and Grow Rich*. Cleveland, OH: Ralston Publishing.

Hollingshead August B. and Fredrick. C. Redlich. 1958. *Social Class and Mental Illness: A Community Study.* New York: Wiley.

Hong Zhaoguang. 2016. "Come to Terms with Yourself – On How to Maintain Psychological Equilibrium." *Secretarial Work* 5 (in Chinese).

Horwitz, Allan V., Helene R. White, and Sandra Howell-White. 1996. "Becoming Married and Mental Health: A Longitudinal Study of a Cohort of Young Adults." *Journal of Marriage and the Family* 58 (November): 895–907.

Hsiao, Fei-Hsiu, Steven Klimidis, Harry Minas, and Eng-Seong Tan. 2006. "Cultural Attribution of Mental Health Suffering in Chinese Societies: The Views of Chinese Patients with Mental Illness and Their Caregivers." *Journal of Clinical Nursing* 15 (8): 998–1006.

Hsu, Francis L. K. 1971. "Psychosocial Homeostasis and Jen: Conceptual Tools for Advancing Psychological Anthropology." *American Anthropologist* 73 (1): 23–44.

Huang, Hsuan-Ying. 2014. "The Emergence of the Psycho-Boom in Contemporary Urban China." In *Psychiatry and Chinese History*, ed. Howard Chiang. London: Pickering & Chatto.

Illouz, Eva. 2007. *Cold Intimacies: The Making of Emotional Capitalism.* Cambridge: Polity.

Illouz, Eva. 2008. *Saving the Modern Soul: Therapy, Emotions, and the Culture of Self-Help.* Berkeley: University of California Press.

Jackson, Todd and Hong Chen. 2007. "Identifying the Eating Disorder Symptomatic in China: The Role of Sociocultural Factors and Culturally Defined Appearance Concerns." *Journal of Psychosomatic Research* 62 (2): 241–9.

Jackson, Todd and Hong Chen. 2008. "Predicting Changes in Eating Disorder Symptoms among Chinese Adolescents: A 9-Month Prospective Study." *Journal of Psychosomatic Research* 64: 87–95.

Jenkins, Janis H. 2011. "Pharmaceutical Self and Imaginary in the Social Field of Psychiatric Treatment." In *Pharmaceutical Self: The Global Shaping of Experience in an Age of Psychopharmacology*, ed. Janis H. Jenkins. Santa Fe, NM: School of Advanced Research Press.

Ji, Fengyuan. 2004. *Linguistic Engineering: Language and Politics in Mao's China.* Honolulu: University of Hawaii Press.

Jiang Han. 2016. "Having Money But Not Wealthy, Why is China's Middle Class Anxious?" WeChat: *Sociology*, July 6 (in Chinese).

Jung, Carl. 1961. *Memories, Dreams, Reflections.* New York: Random House.

Kaiman, Jonathan. 2013. "China Starts to Turn to Drugs as Awareness of Depression Spreads". *Guardian*, November 20. https://www.theguardian.com/world/2013/nov/20/china-depression-antidepressants-drugs.

Kallio, Jyrki. 2011. "Tradition in Chinese Politics." In *FIFA Report*. Helsinki: Finnish Institute of International Affairs.

King, Ambrose Y.C. and Michael H. Bond. 1985. "The Confucian Paradigm of Man: A Sociological View." In *Chinese Culture and Mental Health*, eds. Wen-Shing Tseng and David Y.H. Wu. Orlando, FL: Academic Press.

Kipnis, Andrew B. 1997. *Producing Guanxi: Sentiment, Self and Subculture in a North China Village*. Durham, NC: Duke University Press.

Kipnis, Andrew. 2012. *Chinese Modernity and the Individual Psyche*. New York: Palgrave Macmillan.

Kitanaka, Junko. 2012. *Depression in Japan: Psychiatric Cures for a Society in Distress*. Princeton: Princeton University Press.

Kleinman, Arthur. 1980. *Patients and Healers in the Context of Culture: An Exploration of the Borderland between Anthropology, Medicine, and Psychiatry*. Berkeley: University of California Press.

Kleinman, Arthur. 1986. *Social Origin of Distress and Disease: Depression, Neurasthenia and Pain in Modern China*. New Haven: Yale University Press.

Kleinman, Arthur. 1987. "Anthropology and Psychiatry: The Role of Culture in Cross-Cultural Research on Illness." *British Journal of Psychiatry* 151: 447–54.

Kleinman, Arthur. 1988. *The Illness Narratives: Suffering, Healing and the Human Condition*. New York: Basic Books.

Kleinman, Arthur. 1995. *Writing at the Margin: Discourse between Anthropology and Medicine*. Berkeley: University of California Press.

Kleinman, Arthur. 2009. "Caregiving: The Odyssey of Becoming More Human." *The Lancet* 373 (9660): 292–3.

Kleinman, Arthur. 2010. "The Art of Medicine: Remaking the Moral Person in China: Implications for Health." *The Lancet* 375 (9720): 1074–5.

Kleinman, Arthur and Joan Kleinman. 1991. "Suffering and Its Professional Transformation: Towards an Ethnography of Personal Experience." *Culture, Medicine and Psychiatry* 15: 275–301.

Kleinman, Arthur and Joan Kleinman. 1994. "How Bodies Remember: Social Memory and Bodily Experience of Criticism, Resistance and Delegitimation Following China's Cultural Revolution." *New Literary History* 25: 707–23.

Kleinman, Arthur and Joan Kleinman. 1997. "Moral Transformations of Health and Suffering in Chinese Society." In *Morality and Health*, eds. Allan Brandt and Paul Rozin. New York: Routledge.

Kleinman, Arthur, Yunxiang Yan, Jing Jun, Sing Lee, Everett Zhang, Pan Tianshu, Wu Fei, and Guo Jinhua. 2011. *Deep China: The Moral Life of the Person*. Berkeley: University of California Press.

Komjathy, Louis. 2014. *Daoism: A Guide for the Perplexed*. London and New York: Bloomsbury Academic.

Kuan, Teresa. 2015. *Love's Uncertainty: The Politics and Ethics of Child Rearing in Contemporary China*. Berkeley: University of California Press.

Laing, Ronald. D. 1961. *The Divided Self*. Hamondsworth: Penguin.

Larre, Claude and Rochat de la Vallee. 1996. *The Seventh Emotions: Psychology and Health in Ancient China*. Cambridge: Monkey Press.

Lee, Ching Kwan and Yonghong Zhang. 2013. "The Power of Instability: Unraveling the Microfoundations of Bargained Authoritarianism in China." *American Journal of Sociology* 118 (6): 1475–1508.

Lee, Haiyan. 2007. *Revolution of the Heart: A Genealogy of Love in China, 1900–1950*. Palo Alto, CA: Stanford University Press.

Lee, Sing. 1991. "Anorexia Nervosa in Hong Kong: A Chinese Perspective." *Psychological Medicine* 21 (3): 703–11.

Lee, Sing. 1998. "Higher Earnings, Bursting Trains and Exhausted Bodies: The Creation of Traveling Psychosis in Post-Reform China." *Social Science and Medicine* 47 (9): 1247–61.

Lee, Sing. 2002. "The Stigma of Schizophrenia: A Transcultural Problem." *Current Opinion in Psychiatry* 15 (1): 37–41.

Lee, Sing. 2011. "Depression: Coming of Age in China." In *Deep China: The Moral Life of the Person*, eds. Arthur Kleinman, Yunxiang Yan, Jing Jun, Sing Lee, Everett Zhang, Pan Tianshu, Wu Fei, and Guo Jinhua. Berkeley: University of California Press.

Lee, Sing and Arthur Kleinman. 2003. "Suicide as Resistance in Chinese Society." In *Chinese Society*, ed. Elisabeth Perry. London: Routledge.

Lee, Sing and Antoinette M. Lee. 2000. "Disordered Eating in Three Communities of China: A Comparative Study of Female High School Students in Hong Kong, Shenzhen and Rural Hunan." *International Journal of Eating Disorders* 29: 224–9.

Lee, Sing, Margaret T. Y. Lee, Marcus Y. L. Chiu, and Arthur Kleinman. 2005. "Experience of Social Stigma by People with Schizophrenia in Hong Kong." *The British Journal of Psychiatry* 186 (2): 153–7.

Li, Jie, Juan Li, Graham Thornicroft, and Yuanguang Huang. 2014. "Levels of Stigma among Community Mental Health Staff in Guangzhou, China." *BMC Psychiatry* 14: 231. doi: 10.1186/s12888-014-0231-x.

Li, Lianjiang, Mingxin Liu, and Kevin J. O'Brien. 2012. "Petitioning Beijing: The High Tide of 2003–2006." *The China Quarterly* 210: 313–34.

Li, Shengxian and Michael R. Phillips. 1990. "Witchdoctors and Mental Illness in Mainland China: A Preliminary Study." *American Journal of Psychiatry* 147: 221–4.

Li Zixun. 2016. "Women and Psychology." WeChat: *Li Zixun*, March 16 (in Chinese).

Lin, Yii Nii. 2002. "The Application of Cognitive-Behavioral Therapy to Counseling Chinese." *American Journal of Psychotherapy* 56 (1): 46–58.

Lin Yutang. 1994. *Zhongguoren* [My Country, My People]. Shanghai: Xuelin Chubanshe.

Lin Zuxian. 2016. "The Pathological and Hypocritical Culture of Positive Energy." WeChat: *Si Jian Ke*, August 23 (in Chinese).

Link, Bruce G. and Jo C. Phelan. 2001. "Conceptualizing Stigma." *Annual Review of Sociology* 27: 363–85.

Liu, Jin, Hong Ma, Yan-Ling He, Bin Xie, Yi-Feng Xu, Hong-Yu Tang, Ming Li, Wei Hao, Xiang-Dong Wang, Ming-Yuan Zhang, Chee H. Ng, Margaret Goding, Julia Fraser, Helen Herrman, Helen F.K. Chiu, Sandra S. Chan, Edmond Chiu, and Xin Yu. 2011. "Mental Health System in China: History, Recent Service Reform and Future Challenges." *World Psychiatry* 10: 210–16.

Liu Yiding. 2016. "Locked Mental Patients." *Xin Jing Newspaper*, April 23 (in Chinese).

Liu Yiming. 2014. "Mystery Behind Chinese Officials' Suicides." *Fenghuang Ruiping*, April 16 (in Chinese).

Liu Yuli. 2008. *Xintai Gaibian Mingyun* [Attitude Changes One's Fate]. Beijing: Guojia Xingzheng Xueyuan Yinxiang Chubanshe.

Liu Zhihua. 2012. "Starved for Attention." *China Daily*, September 5 (in Chinese).

Lock, Margaret. 1993. *Encounters with Aging: Mythologies of Menopause in Japan and North America*. Berkeley: University of California Press.

Lu Longguang. 2006. *Xinli Shudao Liaofa* [Psychological Dredging Therapy]. Beijing: The People's Health Press.

Lu, Sunny Y. and Viviana B. Galli. 2002. "Psychiatric Abuse of Falun Gong Practitioners in China." *The Journal of American Academy of Psychiatry and the Law* 30: 126–30.

Luo Dong. 2016. "Chicken Soup for the Soul, a Cup of Aphrodisiac or Coffee?" WeChat: *Ibookreview* (*Xin Jing Bao Shuping Zhoukan*), August 11 (in Chinese).

Lyman, Peter. 2004. "The Domestication of Anger: The Use and Abuse of Anger in Politics." *European Journal of Social Theory* 7 (2): 133–47.

Ma, Zhiying. 2012. "When Love Meets Drugs: Pharmaceuticalizing Ambivalence in Postsocialist China." *Culture, Medicine and Psychiatry* 36: 51–77.

Mao Yushi. 2013. *Zhongguoren de Jiaolv Cong Nali Lai* [Where the Anxiety of the Chinese Came From]. Beijing: Qunyan Chubanshe.

Matthyssen, Mieke. 2012. "*Nande Hutu* and 'the Art of Being Muddled.'" Ph.D. dissertation, University of Ghent.

Matthyssen, Mieke. 2015. "Zheng Banqiao's *Nande Hutu* and 'the Art of Being Muddled' in Contemporary China." *Contemporary Chinese Thought* 46 (4): 3–25.

Matza, Tomas. 2012. "Good Individualism? Psychology, Ethics, and Neoliberalism in Postsocialist Russia." *American Ethnologist* 39 (40): 804–18.

Mbembe, Achille. 2003. "Necropolitics." *Public Culture* 15 (1): 11–40.

McGrath, Jason. 2009. "Communists Have More Fun! The Dialectics of Fulfillment in Cinema of the People's Republic of China." *World Picture* 3. http:// www.worldpicturejournal.com/WP_3/McGrath.html.

Meyer, Donald B. 1980. *Positive Thinkers: Religion as Pop Psychology from Mary Baker Eddy to Oral Roberts* (2nd edn). New York: Pantheon Books.

Miles, Agnes. 1987. *Women and Mental Illness: The Social Context of Female Neurosis*. Brighton: Wheatsheaf Books.

Miller, Peter and Nikolas Rose. 1994. "On Therapeutic Authority: Psychoanalytic Expertise under Advanced Liberalism." *History of the Human Sciences* 7 (30): 29–64.

Miller, Peter and Nikolas Rose. 2008. *Governing the Present: Administering Economic, Social and Personal Life*. Cambridge: Polity.

Mirowsky, John and Catherine E. Ross 2003. *Social Causes of Psychological Distress*. Hawthorne, NY: Aldine de Gruyter.

Moskowitz, Eva S. 2001. *In Therapy We Trust: America's Obsession with Self-Fulfillment*. Baltimore: Johns Hopkins University Press.

Munro, Robin. 2002. *Dangerous Minds: Political Psychiatry in China Today and Its Origins in the Mao Era*. New York: Human Rights Watch and Geneva Initiative on Psychiatry.

Myers, Fred R. 1979. "Emotions and the Self: A Theory of Personhood and Political Order among Pintupi Aborigines." *Ethos* 7 (4): 343–70.

Neitzke, Alex B. 2016. "An Illness of Power: Gender and the Social Causes of Depression." *Culture, Medicine and Psychiatry* 40: 59–73.

Nichter, Mark. 2010. "Idioms of Distress Revisited." *Culture, Medicine and Psychiatry* 34: 401–16.

Nichter, Mark and Jennifer Jo Thompson. 2006. "For My Wellness, Not Just My Illness: North Americans' Use of Dietary Supplements." *Culture, Medicine and Psychiatry* 30: 175–222.

Nolan, James L. 1998. *The Therapeutic State: Justifying Government at Century's End*. New York: New York University Press.

Norwood, Robin. 1985. *Women Who Love Too Much: When You Keep Wishing and Hoping He'll Change*. New York: St. Martin's Press.

O'Brien, Kevin J. and Li Lianjiang. 2006. *Rightful Resistance in Rural China*. Cambridge: Cambridge University Press.

Osburg, John. 2013. *Anxious Wealth: Money and Morality among China's New Rich*. Stanford: Stanford University Press.

Ots, Thomas. 1994. "The Silenced Body – the Expressive *Leib*: On the Dialectic of Mind and Life in the Chinese Cathartic Healing." In *Embodiment and Experience: The Existential Ground of Culture and Self*, ed. Thomas J. Csordas. Cambridge, New York, Melbourne: Cambridge University Press.

Parsons, Talcott. 1965. *Social Structure and Personality*. New York: Free Press.

Patel, Vikram. 2005. "Gender and Mental Health: A Review of Two Textbooks of Psychiatry." *Economic and Political Weekly* 40 (18): 1850–8.

Patel, Vikram and Arthur Kleinman. 2003. "Poverty and Common Mental Disorders in Developing Countries." *Bulletin of the World Health Organization* 81 (8): 609–15.

Patel, Vikram, Ricado Araya, Mauricio de Lima, Ana Ludermir, and Charles Todd. 1999. "Women, Poverty and Common Mental Disorders in Four Restructuring Societies." *Social Science and Medicine* 49 (11): 1461–71.

Pearson, Veronica. 1995. "Goods on Which One Loses: Women and Mental Health in China." *Social Science Medicine* 41: 1159–73.

Pearson, Veronica and Meng Liu. 2002. "Ling's Death: An Ethnography of a Chinese Woman's Suicide." *Suicide and Life-Threatening Behavior* 32 (4): 347–58.

Perry, Elizabeth L. 2002. "Moving the Masses: Emotion Work in the Chinese Revolution." *Mobilization* 7 (2): 111–28.

Phillips, Ari. 2015. "The Smog Blues Descends on China." *Fusion*, December 10. http://tv.fusion.net/story/243898/smog-blues-descends-on-china/.

Phillips, Michael R. 1993. "Strategies Used by Chinese Families Coping with Schizophrenia." In *Chinese Families in the Post-Mao Era*, eds. Deborah Davis and Steven Harrell. Berkeley: University of California Press.

Phillips, Michael R. 2001. "Characteristics, Experience, and Treatment of Schizophrenia in China." *Dialogues in Clinical Neuroscience* 3 (2): 109–19.

Phillips, Michael R. and Veronica Pearson. 1996. "Coping in Chinese Communities: The Need for a New Agenda." In *The Handbook of Chinese Psychology*, ed. Michael H. Bond. Hong Kong: Oxford University Press.

Phillips, Michael R., Zuan Zhao, Xianzhang Xiong, Xiufang Cheng, Guirong Sun, and Ningsheng Wu. 1991. "Changes in the Positive and Negative Symptoms of Hospitalized Schizophrenic Patients in China." *British Journal of Psychiatry* 159: 226–31.

Phillips, Michael R., Charles L. West, Shen Qijie, and Zheng Yanping. 1998. "Comparison of Schizophrenic Patients' Families and Normal Families in China Using Chinese Versions of FACESII and the Family Environment Scales." *Family Process* 37: 95–106.

Phillips, Michael R., Yongyun Li, Scott Stroup, and Lihua Xin. 2000. "Causes of Schizophrenia Reported by Patients' Family Members in China." *British Journal of Psychiatry* 177: 20–5.

Pike, Kathleen M. and Patricia E. Dunne. 2015. "The Rise of Eating Disorders in Asia: A Review." *Journal of Eating Disorders* 3: 33. doi: 10.1186/s40337-015-0070-2.

Polsky, Andrew J. 1991. *The Rise of the Therapeutic State*. Princeton: Princeton University Press.

Potter, Sulamith H. 1988. "The Cultural Construction of Emotion in Rural Chinese Social Life." *Ethos* 16 (2): 181–208.

Pritzker, Sonya E. 2016. "New Age with Chinese Characteristics? Translating Inner Child Emotion Pedagogies in Contemporary China." *Ethos* 44 (2): 150–70.

Pupavac. Vanessa. 2001. "Therapeutic Governance: Psycho-social Intervention and Trauma Risk Management." *Disasters* 25 (4): 358–72.

Pupavac, Vanessa. 2005. "Human Security and the Rise of Global Therapeutic Governance." *Conflict, Security and Development* 5(2): 161–81.

Qi Xingfa. 2013. "Collective Corruption, External Pressure, and Worsened Political Ecology: A Political Scientific Analysis of Officials' Suicide During the Transitional Period." *Theory and Reform* 5 (in Chinese). http://comments.caijing.com.cn/2013-11-28/113624310.html .

Qian, Jiwei. 2012. "Mental Health Care in China: Providing Services for Undertreated Patients." *Journal of Mental Health Policy and Economics* 15(4): 179–86.

Qian, Mingyi, Craig W. Smith, Zhonggeng Chen, and Guohua Xia. 2002. "Psychotherapy in China: A Review of Its History and Contemporary Directions." *International Journal of Mental Health* 30 (4): 49–68.

Qin, Xuezheng, Wang Suyin and Chee-Ruey Hsieh. 2015. "The Prevalence of Depression and Depressive Symptoms among Adults in China: Estimation Based on a National Household Survey." https://editorialexpress.com/cgi-bin/conference/download.cgi?db_name=WCCE2015&paper_id=117.

Rocca, Jean-Louis. 2003. "Old Working Class, New Working Class: Reforms, Labor Crisis and the Two Faces of Conflicts in Chinese Urban Areas." In *China Today: Economic Reforms, Social Cohesion and Collective Identities*, eds. Taciana Fisac and Leila Fernandez-Stembridge. London and New York: RoutledgeCurzon.

Rofel, Lisa. 1999. *Other Modernities: Gendered Yearnings in China after Socialism*. Berkeley: University of California Press.

Rofel, Lisa. 2007. *Desiring China: Experiments in Neoliberalism, Sexuality, and Public Culture*. Durham, NC: Duke University Press.

Rose, Nikolas. 1996. *Inventing Our Selves: Psychology, Power and Personhood.* Cambridge: Cambridge University Press.

Rose, Nikolas. 2006. *The Politics of Life Itself: Biomedicine, Power, and Subjectivity in the Twenty-First Century.* Princeton, NJ: Princeton University Press.

Rose, Nikolas and Joelle M. Abi-Rached. 2013. *Neuro: The New Brain Sciences and the Management of the Mind.* Princeton: Princeton University Press.

Russell, Gerald. 2000. "Anorexia Nervosa." In *New Oxford Textbook of Psychiatry*, eds. Michael Gelder, Nancy Andreasen, Juan Lopez-Ibor, and John Geddes. New York: Oxford University Press.

Sapio, Flora. 2008. "*Shuanggui* and Extralegal Detention in China." *China Information* 22 (1): 7–37.

Sampson, Edward E. 1981. "Cognitive Psychology as Ideology." *American Psychologist* 36: 730–43.

Shao Jingjun. 2016. "Psychological Health Should Become an Important Criterion for Appointing Cadres." *Chinese Cadres Tribune* 3: 16–18 (in Chinese).

Shapiro, Francine and Deany Laliotis. 2010. "EMDR and the Adaptive Information Processing Model: Integrative Treatment and Case Conceptualization." *Clinical Social Work Journal* 39 (2): 191–200.

Shi, Tianjian. 2015. *The Cultural Logic of Politics in Mainland China and Taiwan.* New York: Cambridge University Press.

Shi, Tianjian and Jie Lu. 2010a. "The Shadow of Confucianism." *Journal of Democracy* 21 (4): 123–30.

Shi, Tianjian and Jie Lu. 2010b. "Cultural Impacts on People's Understanding of Democracy." Paper presented at the 2010 American Political Science Association Annual Meeting, Washington, DC, September 1–5.

Shun, Kwong-loi. 2011. "On Anger: An Experimental Essay in Confucian Moral Psychology." In *Zhu Xi Now: Contemporary Encounters with the Great Ultimate*, eds. David Jones and He Jinli. Albany: State University of New York Press.

Solinger, Dorothy. 2006. "The Creation of a New Underclass in China and its Implications." *Environment and Urbanization* 18 (1): 177–93.

Sundararajan, Louise. 2015. *Understanding Emotion in Chinese Culture: Thinking Through Psychology.* New York: Springer.

Sundararajan, Louise. 2016. "Rebuttal to Jahoda on IP." *Indigenous Psychology Listserv*, July 5, http://indigenouspsych.org/Discussion/forum/PDF/Rebuttal%20to%20Jahoda%20on%20IP.pdf.

Szasz, Thomas S. 1963. *Law, Liberty, and Psychiatry: An Inquiry into the Social Uses of Mental Health Practices.* New York: Macmillan.

Tang Yinghong. 2016. "Treating Internet Addiction with ECT is Like Curing Habitual Masturbation by Cutting Off One's Hands." WeChat: *PsyEyes.* August 21 (in Chinese).

Thornicroft, Graham, Diana Rose, Aliya Kassam, and Norman Sartorius. 2007. "Stigma: Ignorance, Prejudice or Discrimination?" *British Journal of Psychiatry* 190: 192–3.

Townsend, John M and Cynthia L. Carbone. 1980. "Menopausal Syndrome: Illness or Social Role – A Transcultural Analysis." *Culture, Medicine and Psychiatry* 4 (3): 229–48.

Vannoy Steven. D. and William. T. Hoyt. 2004. "Evaluation of an Anger Therapy Intervention for Incarcerated Adult Males". *Journal of Offender Rehabilitation* 39 (2): 39–52.

Walder, Andrew G. 1986. *Communist Neo-Traditionalism: Work and Authority in Chinese Industry*. Berkeley: University of California Press.

Wang Dingding. 2016. "What Will Happen in Beijing under Long-Term Smog." January10 (in Chinese). http://scholarsupdate.hi2net.com/news.asp?NewsID=19164.

Wang Xiaodong. 2017. "First Guideline Issued on Improving Mental Health." *China Daily*, January 19. http://www.chinadaily.com.cn/china/2017-01/19/content_28002875.htm.

Wang Xiaoyu. 2016. "What is More Terrible Than Smog is Yu Dan; What is More Terrible Than Yu Dan is Jitang." WeChat: *Qiangwai Naxieshi'er*. October 10 (in Chinese).

Wang, Xin. 2014. "In Pursuit of Status: The Rising Consumerism of China's Middle Class." In *The Changing Landscape of China's Consumerism*, ed. Alison Hulme. Oxford: Elsevier.

Wang Xiuqiu. 2008. *Ganbian Qianwan Ren Yisheng de Xinli Jianya Fa* [The Psychological De-stressing Practices that Benefit All]. Haikou, Hainan Province: Nanhai Shubanshe.

Wang, Zheng. 2003. "Gender, Employment and Women's Resistance." In *Chinese Society: Change, Conflict and Resistance*, eds. Elizabeth J. Perry and Mark Selden. New York: Routledge Curzon.

WHO. 2002. "Gender and Mental Health – World Health Organization." http://apps.who.int/iris/bitstream/10665/68884/1/a85573.pdf.

Wills, Frank. 2010. *Skills in Cognitive Behavior Counseling and Psychotherapy*. London: Sage.

Wright, Steven, Andrew Day, and Kevin Howells. 2009. "Mindfulness and the Treatment of Anger Problems." *Aggression and Violent Behavior* 14 (5): 396–401.

Wu, Fei. 2010. *Suicide and Justice: A Chinese Perspective*. Abingdon: Routledge.

Wu Si. 2001. *Qian Guize: Zhongguo Lishi de Zhenshi Youxi* [Hidden Rules: The True Games of Chinese History]. Kunming: Yunnan People's Press.

Wu Xi'an. 2016. "The Stronger the Mother is, the More She Will Be Detrimental to the Family." WeChat: *Philosophical Life Net*, July 23 (in Chinese).

Wu Zhihong. 2016. *Juying Guo* [Nation of Giant Infants]. Hangzhou: Zhejiang People's Publishing House.

Xia Yufen, Song Tingsheng, Zheng Zhanpei, Wang Defang, Fu Guozhen, Zhou Sheng, Yu Weiyuan, and Zhu Weibing. 1990. "Changes in Delusional Content in Paranoid Schizophrenia in China." *Shanghai Archives of Psychiatry* 3: 133–7 (in Chinese).

Xia Mianzun. 1926. "Thoughts on a Folk Ballad." *Xin Nüxing* 7: 62–7 (in Chinese).

Xiao Lou Laoshi. 2016. "How Does a Poisonous Mother–Daughter Relationship Affect the Daughter's Life?" WeChat: *Yi Xinlin*, September 19 (in Chinese).

Xu Kaiwen. 2016. "Empty Heart Disease of This Era – the Disaster of China's Utilitarian Exam-centered Education." July 19 (in Chinese). http://zhuanlan. zhihu.com/p/21651116.

Yan, Yunxiang. 1996. "The Culture of *Guanxi* in a North China Village." *The China Journal* 35: 1–25.

Yan, Yunxiang. 2011. "The Changing Moral Landscape." In *Deep China: The Moral Life of the Person*, eds. Arthur Kleinman, Yunxiang Yan, Jing Jun, Sing Lee, Everett Zhang, Pan Tianshu, Wu Fei, and Guo Jinhua. Berkeley: University of California Press.

Yang, Jie. 2007. "'Reemployment Stars': Language, Gender and Neoliberal Restructuring in China." In *Words, Worlds, Material Girls: Language, Gender and Global Economies*, ed. Bonnie McElhinny. Berlin: Mouton de Gruyter.

Yang, Jie. 2010. "The Crisis of Masculinity: Class, Gender and Kindly Power in Post-Mao China." *American Ethnologist* 37 (3): 550–62.

Yang, Jie. 2011a. "The Politics of the Dang'an: Spectralization, Spatialization, and Neoliberal Governmentality in China." *Anthropological Quarterly* 84 (2): 507–34.

Yang, Jie. 2011b. "*Nennu* and *Shunu*: Gender, Body Politics and the Beauty Economy in China." *Signs: Journal of Women in Culture and Society* 36 (2): 333–57.

Yang, Jie. 2013. "Fake Happiness: Counseling, Potentiality and Psycho-politics in China." *Ethos* 41 (3): 291–311.

Yang, Jie. 2014. "The Happiness of the Marginalized: Affect, Counseling and Self-Reflexivity in China." In *The Political Economy of Affect and Emotion in East Asia*, ed. Jie Yang. Abingdon and New York: Routledge.

Yang, Jie. 2015. *Unknotting the Heart: Unemployment and Therapeutic Governance in China*. Ithaca, NY: Cornell University Press.

Yang, Jie. 2016. "The Politics and Regulation of Anger in Urban China." *Culture, Medicine and Psychiatry* 41: 100–23.

Yang, Jie. 2017. "Virtuous Power: Ethics, Confucianism and Psychological Self-Help in China." *Critique of Anthropology*. doi.org/10.1177/03082 75X17694943.

Yang, Jie. Forthcoming. "Happy Housewives: Gender, Class and Psychological Self-Help in Urban China." In *Chinese Discourses on Happiness*, eds. Gerda Wielander and Derek Hird. Hong Kong: Hong Kong University Press.

Yang, Lawrence Hsin. 2007. "Application of Mental Illness Stigma Theory to Chinese Societies: Synthesis and New Directions." *Singapore Medical Journal* 48 (11): 977–85.

Yang, Lawrence Hsin and Arthur Kleinman. 2008. "'Face' and the Embodiment of Stigma in China: The Cases of Schizophrenia and AIDS." *Social Science & Medicine* 67 (3): 398–408.

Yang, Lawrence Hsin, Arthur Kleinman, Bruce G. Link, Jo C. Phelan, Sing Lee, and Byron Good. 2007. "Culture and Stigma: Adding Moral Experience to Stigma Theory." *Social Science & Medicine* 64: 1524–35.

Yang, Mayfair Meihui. 1999. *Spaces of Their Own: Women's Public Sphere in Transnational China*. Minneapolis: University of Minnesota Press.

Yang Yang. 2015. "A Simple Way to Treat the Epidemic of Buying Things." *China Daily*, November 11. http://europe.chinadaily.com.cn/culture/2015-11/11/content_22424708.htm.

Yarris, Kristin Elizabeth. 2014 "'Pensando Mucho' ('Thinking Too Much'): Embodied Distress among Grandmothers in Nicaraguan Transnational Families." *Culture, Medicine and Psychiatry* 38: 473–98.

Yu Dan. 2006. *Lunyu Xinde* [Yu Dan's Interpretation of the *Analects*]. Beijing: Zhonghua Shuju.

Yu Ying. 2011. "Heart-pleasing Electronics." *Xinli Yuekan* 62: 120 (in Chinese).

Yu Yongjie. 2016. "Filtering Mental Diseases: Do Not Offer Wrong Prescription." WeChat: *Tuanjiehu Cankao*, August 4 (in Chinese).

Yuen, Lotus. 2013. "Unable to Cope: China's Inadequate Care of the Mentally Ill." *The Atlantic*, July 29. http://www.theatlantic.com/china/archive/2013/07/unable-to-cope-chinas-inadequate-care-of-the-mentally-ill/278170/.

Zha, Rui. 2016. "Report, I Found One Mentally Ill Person." WeChat: *Shanghai Observations*, July 22 (in Chinese).

Zhang, Amy Y., Lucy C. Yu, Jianping Yuan, Zhifu Tong, Chaoyuan Yang and Stephen E. Foreman. 1997. "Family and Cultural Correlates of Depression among Chinese Elders". *International Journal of Social Psychiatry* 43 (3): 199–212.

Zhang Defen. 2016. "Women, the Force to Change the World, Begin with You Yourself" – A Speech at "Her Village International Forum." WeChat: *Tefenchangpublic*, August 23 (in Chinese).

Zhang, Jin. 2014. "Who Are More Prone to Develop Depression?" WeChat: *Caixinwang*, May 12 (in Chinese).

Zhang, Jin. 2016. "Treatment Relies on Hospitals and Recovery on Community." WeChat: *Duguo*, December 7 (in Chinese).

Zhang, Li. 2014. "Bentuhua: Culturing Psychotherapy in Postsocialist China". *Culture, Medicine and Psychiatry* 38: 283–305.

Zhang, Li. 2015. "Cultivating Happiness: Psychotherapy, Spirituality, and Well-Being in a Transforming Urban China." In *Handbook of Religion and the Asian City: Aspiration and Urbanization in the Twenty-First Century*, ed. Peter van der Veer. Berkeley: University of California Press.

Zhang, Li. 2017. "The Rise of Therapeutic Governing in Postsocialist China." *Medical Anthropology* 36 (1): 6–18.

Zhang, Li and Aihwa Ong. 2008. *Privatizing China: Socialism from Afar*. Ithaca, NY: Cornell University Press.

Zhang, Tong and Barry Schwartz. 1997. "Confucius and the Cultural Revolution: A Study in Collective Memory." *International Journal of Politics, Culture and Society* 11(2): 189–212.

Zhang, Yalin, Derson Young, Sing Lee, Honggen Zhang, Zeping Xiao, Wei Hao, Yongmin Feng, Hongxiang Zhou, and Doris F. Chang. 2002. "Chinese Taoist Cognitive Psychotherapy in the Treatment of Generalized Anxiety Disorder in Contemporary China." *Transcultural Psychiatry* 34: 115–29.

Zhang, Yanhua. 2007. *Transforming Emotions through Chinese Medicine: An Ethnographic Account from Contemporary China*. Albany: State University of New York Press.

Zhang, Yanhua. 2014. "Crafting Confucian Remedies for Happiness in Contemporary China: Unraveling the Yu Dan Phenomenon." In *The Political Economy of Affect and Emotion in East Asia*, ed. Jie Yang, London and New York: Routledge.

Zheng, Jun. 2009. *Xinli Zhuren de Di San Shili* [The Third Force of Psychological Self-Help]. Shanghai: Chinese Northeast Normal University Press.

Zhou Guoping. 2016. *Chengzhang Shi Jian Gudu de Shi* [Growing Up is Lonely]. Beijing: Zhongguo Qingnian Chubanshe.

Zhou Xiaohong. 2014. "Anxiety: The Epochal Symptom of Rapid Social Changes." *Jiangsu Xingzheng Xueyuan Xuebao* 6: 54–7 (in Chinese).

Zhu Jianjun. 2008. *Laizi Dongfang de Xinli Liaofa: Yixiang Duihua Xinli Zhiliao* [Psychotherapy from the Orient: Imagery Communication Psychotherapy]. Beijing: Beijing Daxue Yixue Chubanshe (in Chinese with English translation).

# Index

United States, 2, 10, 181, 182, 183
university students, 71–3

values
adjusting, 25
Chinese cultural tradition, 9, 16
Communist Party, 9
Confucianism, 17, 86, 105, 155–6, 161, 211
video game addiction, 49, 51
video surveillance, 136
violence, patients, 126–8
virtue, 195–200

Wang Dingding, 56
Wang Jian, 56–7
Wang Xiaoxing, 186
Wang Xiaoyu, 186
Watson, Amy, 116
WeChat, 18, 158
*wei xingfu* (fake happiness), 191–2
Weibo (microblog), 32
Wen Jiabao, 6
Western approaches
Chinese practice, 25, 35
Chinese vs. Western approaches, 4, 9, 27, 210
cognitive therapy, 155, 160
critics, 173
dominance, 131
hybridizing, 178, 206
inadequacy in China, 48
indigenous psychology and, 157–61
infiltration, 156
legitimizing, 212
patients' autonomy, 30–1
privilegization of emotions, 38–9
psychological dredging therapy and, 164

self-help, 181–2
therapeutic governance, 16
winter blues, 57
women
beauty, 78, 96
depression, 81–2, 86–7
eating disorders, 78
economic restructuring and, 76–8
exploitation, 22
happiness and, 187
incidence of mental illness, 75, 81
mothers, 80–1, 85–91
negative social situation, 76
obedience and submission, 86
other-orientation, 86
pathologizing, 22
mothers, 85–91
professional women, 79
roles, 78–72
self-help, 182, 186
social exclusion, 22
socioeconomics and, 98, 209–10
suicides, 86, 87
thinness cult, 94–6
unemployment, 76, 88–9
violence against, 87, 88
work unit system, 65–6
workaholics, 73
World Health Organization, 2, 102, 113, 131
World Mental Health Day, 207
Wu Si, 44
Wu Xi'an, 80–1
Wu Zhihong, 93, 158, 170–3
*wuwei* (non-action, not-forcing), 166, 168

Xi Jinping, 46
Xia Mianzun, 182, 186
Xia Yufen, 132